Adult Interpersonal Violence

This unique volume uses an occupational perspective to shine a light on how the impact of interpersonal violence (IPV) affects people in their daily tasks and activities.

The book recognises how the legacy of trauma – whether it be from one or more events that were physically, verbally, emotionally, sexually, or psychologically harmful or threatening – can be seen in the occupational experiences of both victims/survivors and perpetrators. It fills a distinct gap in the literature and highlights a pervasive issue – one which occupational therapists must regularly contend with. Edited by a leading scholar from both the United States and the United Kingdom and including chapters on IPV within intimate relationships, stalking, and sexual assault, the book takes the field of occupational therapy into a new direction, setting the research agenda as well as, through invaluable clinical guidance, informing professional practice.

This book will be essential reading for students, scholars, and practitioners across the field of occupational science and occupational therapy.

Rebecca (Bex) Twinley is a part-time senior lecturer in occupational therapy at the University of Brighton, England, UK, and works part-time in practice in neurodevelopmental services.

Christine Helfrich is a professor in the Division of Occupational Therapy at American International College, Massachusetts, USA.

Adult Interpersonal Violence

Illuminating the Dark Side of Occupations

Edited by Rebecca Twinley and Christine Helfrich

Routledge
Taylor & Francis Group
LONDON AND NEW YORK

First published 2025
by Routledge
4 Park Square, Milton Park, Abingdon, Oxon OX14 4RN

and by Routledge
605 Third Avenue, New York, NY 10158

Routledge is an imprint of the Taylor & Francis Group, an informa business

British Library Cataloguing-in-Publication Data
A catalogue record for this book is available from the British Library

ISBN: 978-1-032-72685-4 (hbk)
ISBN: 978-1-032-72686-1 (pbk)
ISBN: 978-1-032-72687-8 (ebk)

DOI: 10.4324/9781032726878

Typeset in Times New Roman
by Apex CoVantage, LLC

This book is dedicated to the memory of Mel (QC) Joyner. I miss you, with love and appreciation from your non-biological daughter. I am also privileged to dedicate this book to my daughter: your safety and happiness in this world mean absolutely everything to me.

Bex Twinley

This book is dedicated to my daughter, Olivia. May you live in a world where women and girls do not have to experience the shame of interpersonal violence.

Christine Helfrich

Contents

Contributors

Sam Baker is a lecturer in occupational therapy at the University of Liverpool, England, UK.

Christine Helfrich is a professor in the Division of Occupational Therapy at American International College, Massachusetts, USA.

Kim Jones is the occupational therapy lead of Adult Mental Health Team at Betsi Cadwaladr University Health Board, Wrexham, Wales, UK.

Rebecca (Bex) Twinley is a part-time senior lecturer in occupational therapy at the University of Brighton, England, UK, and works part-time in practice in neurodevelopmental services.

Figures

Tables

Preface

Bex

On November 9, 2022, Russell George, an editor for Routledge I had formerly worked with, emailed me to update me on sales of the (first) book I edited, *Illuminating the Dark Side of Occupation: International Perspectives from Occupational Therapy and Occupational Science* (Twinley, 2021). Russell asked if I had any further writing or editing plans, proposing the potential scope for an international handbook in the area of the dark side of occupation (this could still happen, Russell). Recognising I had only recently completed editing on this significant project, he also suggested, alternatively, producing a book for their short-form series, called Routledge Focus. On November 22, 2022, I wrote back about my preceding ideas for a text that presents an occupational perspective of interpersonal violence, and it was at this point that my hopes and thoughts on this topic surged and intensified, and subsequent to having co-edited this text, they have necessarily evolved. By referring to an 'occupational perspective', I adopt Njelesani et al.'s definition as being a "way of looking at or thinking about human doing" (2014, p. 226); this lens and knowledge of occupations are influenced by personal and contextual factors (Laliberte Rudman et al., 2022).

I value my profession as an occupational therapist. However, my growth and development as an occupational therapist and, later, as an occupational scientist have been greatly shaped and characterised by my critical thinking, which – in turn – has shaped my own occupational perspective; I see this as grounded in my personality traits and personally held values of fairness, justice, intellectual integrity, being reasonable, and a love of learning – all of which I largely attribute to (a) being a victim/survivor who has experienced much trauma, pain, blame, and dehumanisation and (b) being autistic and ADHD and understanding these traits as core character strengths. Critical and reflective thinking has become a fundamental skill that I utilise in my practice as an occupational therapist, as an occupational therapy lecturer (educator), and as an occupational therapy and occupational science researcher, scholar, colleague, and critic. More than anything, this critical and reflective thinking has fostered my articulation of a perceived need for innovation, improvement, and genuine change, especially given my reflections on the limitations, inadequacies, and opportunities within the professional body of literature pertaining to occupations.

In December 2022, after Allison Sullivan had kindly introduced Chris and me via email, I wrote to Chris to propose my idea and to invite her to join me to co-edit this book. In this email, I explained:

> I would really like to highlight the work occupational therapists are doing (and therefore can do) in the broad are of interpersonal violence with some specific examples. . . . Given the legacy I feel you have left the profession in seeking to explore this under-addressed/explored area (hence, falls within remit of my concept of the dark side of occupation), I am writing to you to see if you would consider co-editing with myself.
>
> (R. Twinley, personal communication, December 7, 2022)

Almost a year on from Russell's email, on October 11, 2023, Chris and I signed the contract for this text. It was so important to me to capture and share occupational perspectives of working with people impacted by interpersonal violence from colleagues who have had experience in their occupational therapy practice. Chris and I are honoured and grateful to have Sam and Kim as occupational therapy colleagues who joined us on this venture and who offer just this. There is much need for theory to be applied in practice to 'test it out' and for individuals to develop their own professional identity. Sam and Kim's chapters promote their unique contributions as occupational therapists in the teams with whom they worked.

In terms of the audience and relevance of this text, Chris and I identified the most likely readers and users of this book would be those from the disciplines of occupational therapy and occupational science, alongside those in public health, trauma studies, psychology, criminology, allied health, and social work. We envisaged the primary market would be the following:

- Educators (academics) and researchers
- Occupational therapy practitioners (across a range of settings – not just mental health)
- Occupational scientists (which is interdisciplinary and so attracts a range of disciplines and professions to its readership)
- Post-professional occupational therapy/occupational science students
- Students at all pre-registration education levels (BSc through to post-doctoral)

Having completed editing its contents, I additionally strongly feel that this book has importance for victims/survivors of interpersonal violence. I hope reading the stories contained assists with dissipating any feelings of loneliness and isolation. In the same tone that I end the final chapter, I also hope you take encouragement from the fact there are occupational therapy practitioners who are both contributing to (participating in) and commanding the transformation and development of service response and provision. I am certainly grateful to those who are taking on this difficult, demanding, emotion work.

Chris

My career as an occupational therapist has always been filled with questions about the ideas and practices of the profession. Even as an entry-level bachelor's student, I questioned everything. As a clinician, I questioned the assumptions espoused by our theoretical frameworks. In fact, my master's thesis with Gary Kielhofner as my advisor challenged his conceptualisation of the volition subsystem in the Model of Human Occupation and resulted in its revision to focus on narrative and understanding the meaning of therapy (Kielhofner et al., 1995). Since then, I have continued to understand the experiences and meaning of occupations to what has been referred to as 'marginalised populations', primarily those who have experienced domestic violence and those who are unhoused, including the various subpopulations that comprise these groups. While much of this work has been framed within occupational science, I believe the dark side of occupation would have been a pivotal tool for further illumination.

Bex and Chris

In terms of what to expect in this book, the content is about interpersonal violence, which may be physical, sexual, or psychological and includes rape, sexual assault, intimate partner (dating or relationship) violence, and stalking. Acts of interpersonal violence are further divided into family or intimate partner violence (occurring within the family or between intimate partners) and community violence (occurring among individuals not related by family connections but who may or may not know each other). Globally, interpersonal violence is a pervasive public health, human rights, economics, and development challenge. In all its forms, the perpetration of interpersonal violence between adults cannot be denied, with the COVID-19 global pandemic only highlighting and exacerbating its prevalence in our communities.

In this book, we explore positionality and reflexivity. As a writing team, we are occupational therapists who – in our roles as either practitioner or researcher – have all had contact with victims/survivors of interpersonal violence, yet we remain cognisant of the paucity of research related to the occupational therapy role within our professional literature. We argue for an occupational perspective of interpersonal violence that understands the incidence between adults can be experienced by any person in any setting and spans the intersections of age, class, culture, disability, ethnicity, gender identity, migration status, place of residence, race, religion, sex, sexual orientation, and socioeconomic status. Case vignettes are presented as a way to support the information provided and to give case examples; however, these have the potential to stir responses in some readers, considering they are all focused on traumatic events. Overall, this is an essential read that illuminates the impact of interpersonal violence; identifies key recommendations; and elucidates the occupational therapy role for practitioners, scholars, educators, and students who are either knowingly or unknowingly working with or alongside victims/survivors.

References

Kielhofner, G., Borell, L., Burke, J., Helfrich, C.A., & Nygard, L. (1995). Volition subsystem. In G. Kielhofner (Ed.), *A model of human occupation: Theory and application* (2nd ed., pp. 39–62). Williams & Wilkins.

Laliberte Rudman, D., Aldrich, R., & Kiepek, N. (2022). Evolving understandings of occupation. In M. Egan & G. Restall (Eds.), *Promoting occupational participation: Collaborative relationship-focused occupational therapy* (pp. 11–30). Canadian Association of Occupational Therapists.

Njelesani, J., Tang, A., Jonsson, H., & Polatajko, H. (2014). Articulating an occupational perspective. *Journal of Occupational Science*, *21*(2), 226–235. https://doi.org/10.1080/14427591.2012.717500

Twinley, R. (Ed.). (2021). *Illuminating the dark side of occupation: International perspectives from occupational therapy and occupational science.* Routledge. https://doi.org/10.4324/9780429266256

Acknowledgements

Thanks to those people who, earlier on in my adult life, helped me in some way or to some extent to feel heard, able to tell (some of) my story, and the stories of others. Some of you are now gone, but this includes Mel (QC) Joyner, Gayle Letherby, Marj Dawson, Alyss T, S. Caroline Taylor, Graham Sewell, and, more recently, Sharon Y.

I would like to express my ongoing gratitude to the respondents of my doctoral study and to those victims/survivors who reach out and contact me, often in times of loneliness and hopelessness; your ability and willingness to share your experiences, your stories, are forever appreciated.

For helping bring this book to fruition and to illuminate these hard topics and issues, I am grateful to Chris (Helfrich), Sam Baker, Kim Jones, Russell George, and Allison Sullivan.

Rebecca (Bex) Twinley

Thanks to those people who supported my questioning the status quo in occupational therapy and encouraged me to challenge and critique the profession with innovative ideas. This includes professors John Bazyk, Gary Kielhofner, David Beer, and Anne Fischer; my colleagues Simone Gill, Wendy Hildenbrand, Susan Haiman, and Linda Learnard; and my students who helped me grow and learn through their critiques and questions, especially Ann Aviles de Bradley and Emily Simpson. I must also acknowledge the staff of the National Institute for Independent Living, Rehabilitation and Research (NIDILRR) for recognising the importance of funding research to understand the experience of domestic violence so necessary to developing interventions. Most importantly, I thank Joyce Cowan and the staff of Family Rescue, Inc., for mentoring me and providing me access to their clients – women and children who experienced domestic violence. These individuals and others who shared their stories with me are the true heroes of this work; without them, nothing would have been accomplished. Finally, I thank Allison Sullivan for connecting me with Bex, and Bex, Sam, and Kim for their personal and professional support and collaboration over these past three years.

Christine Helfrich

1 What's illuminating the dark side of occupation got to do with it?

Christine Helfrich

A note to readers

There are many ethical issues related to the research and preparation of the content within the following chapters. This includes the importance of content warnings (rather than problematic 'trigger' warnings) necessary to forewarn readers that some content may be sensitive or emotionally provocative and may activate a response you find overwhelming or that you weren't expecting. We encourage you to prepare before reading and to make use of strategies to lessen or avoid any harm that could occur as an outcome of reading any traumatic or difficult material. We also acknowledge those readers who have experienced vicarious trauma and compassion fatigue when working in practice to support victims/survivors or perpetrators of interpersonal violence.

Introduction

The dark side of occupation is an emerging concept in the occupational therapy and occupational science literature (Twinley, 2021). It is also not the only way in which to view or try to understand and conceptualise the complexities of occupations. Its focus in these chapters is clarified and discussed. This chapter will present the theoretical premise for discussing experiences related to surviving and perpetuating interpersonal violence as occupations that are not well understood or embraced within the occupational therapy profession. Each chapter thereafter will present groundbreaking practice or research in occupational therapy/occupational science that was completed by the author. Specifically, Kim Jones introduces the first programme that included occupational therapy with women who are victims/survivors of domestic violence in the United Kingdom, while Sam Baker presents the role of occupational therapy in the rehabilitation of stalkers, also in the United Kingdom. Rebecca (Bex) Twinley discusses her qualitative research with women from various countries who have experienced woman-to-woman rape and sexual assault. Lastly, Bex and I conclude this text with a discussion of future directions for occupational therapy and occupational science.

DOI: 10.4324/9781032726878-1

As a writing team, we are occupational therapists who – in our roles as practitioners, academics, or researchers – have had contact with victims/survivors of interpersonal violence, yet we remain cognisant of the paucity of research related to the occupational therapy role within our professional literature. Given interpersonal violence is a major global public health problem (World Health Organization [WHO], 2024a), we argue for an occupational perspective that understands that incidents between adults can be experienced by anyone in any setting and spans the intersections of age, class, culture, disability, ethnicity, gender identity, migration status, place of residence, race, religion, sex, sexual orientation, and socioeconomic status. This calls for perspectives that scrutinise the inherent complex dynamics of interpersonal violence to gain a deeper understanding from an occupational perspective.

This book illuminates both the impact of interpersonal violence and the role of occupational therapy for practitioners, scholars, educators, and students who are either knowingly or unknowingly working with or alongside victims/survivors.

When Rebecca (Bex) Twinley contacted me to discuss the proposal for this book, I wasn't quite sure what to expect or how I might respond. I only knew of the *Dark Side of Occupation* as it had been described to me as "the book about 'dark occupations'". When I heard that Bex wanted to write a book about 'interpersonal violence and the dark side of occupations', I felt it was my professional responsibility to, at a minimum, listen and understand what she was planning to do. I felt protective of the discussion of the role of occupational therapy with domestic violence and was concerned that I might not approve of her intended portrayal.

Before our first Transatlantic Zoom meeting, I did my due diligence to learn about 'the dark side' and found that what I had been told did not match what Rebecca (Bex) Twinley and others had written (e.g. Twinley, 2021). Still, I was nervous about the first meeting and anticipated it would be challenging. To my surprise and relief, the initial meeting was delightful and changed my own paradigm of how I would further view, conceptualise, and discuss the dark side of occupations. The framework of 'the dark side of occupations' provides a vocabulary and language to understand and describe many of the occupations that, for instance, silenced, ignored, or marginalised individuals engage in daily. I realised that the dark side of occupation was the perfect way to frame most of what I have studied throughout my career and left the meeting wondering how much easier it would have been to communicate with others if I'd had this language 35 years ago! We discussed the collaborators Bex had lined up to write chapters – both Kim Jones and Sam Baker had connected with Bex because her use of the dark side of occupations provided them with a framework for understanding their populations of interest in practice (domestic violence and stalking, respectively), and they were eager to share their work more broadly.

We decided that as the non-coiner of the 'dark side of occupation' concept, it made sense for me to write this introduction from the perspective of a 'dark side of occupation' student and convert. The process of further study and discussion with others has been illuminating. First, I learned that Bex has found that the concept has been well received outside of occupational therapy or occupational science by colleagues in psychology, sociology, and criminology. As Bex discusses in Chapter 4, she actually developed her early ideas through working with a criminologist, and so its early conceptualisation was focused upon their mutual scholarly interests in criminal and 'antisocial' occupations. Hence, our aim to offer some exploration of interpersonal violence from an occupational perspective means to offer "a way of looking at or thinking about human doing" (Njelesani et al., 2014, p. 226) within the remit of this public health issue.

I have become very proficient at describing the metaphor Twinley created to illustrate her framework. The 'dark side' of occupations is like the dark side of the moon – the parts that we cannot see. Or, as with occupations, I would argue it is the occupations that we *choose* not to see, or it is those people we cannot discuss because the necessary conditions for this are not enabled or created. Bex has previously elucidated: " 'the dark side of occupation' is figurative language pointing to the systematic lack of attention and exploration given to certain classes of occupations that have, therefore, been left in the dark" (Twinley, 2021, p. 3). These include the occupations that are not viewed as attractive or related to well-being. In fact, in the context of this text, they are the occupations that are often associated with shame, disgust, blame, embarrassment, and humiliation. Some are illegal or not socially accepted by people's respective local cultures or their society, while others reflect being in the role of victim or being powerless. Illuminating the dark side of occupations requires open discussion and acknowledgement of activities and occupations that many victims/survivors subjectively experience, yet practitioners, faculty, and researchers would seemingly either prefer to ignore these or can find it challenging to initiate discussion of them. Notably, those of us that study/work in the world of these occupations are often faced with the same negative response from our colleagues, family, friends, and students. It is not uncommon to be asked questions such as 'What does this have to do with occupational therapy/occupational science?', 'How did you get stuck with that topic?', and 'Who is making you study that? – Are you the newest faculty member/student so you got what was left to study/teach?' Of course, for those of us who choose to do this work, the answer is 'no'. In fact, we are energised by understanding and learning about these occupations, despite the tremendous burden of doing so.

The challenge of working within the dark side of occupations (as it pertains to those associated with interpersonal violence) includes considering one's own physical/emotional health and safety, being accountable for using trauma-informed approaches to avoid doing further harm – all while owning the important responsibility of educating others why it is so critically important for occupational therapists/scientists to study and understand interpersonal violence. By trauma-informed, I mean working in ways that reduce the adverse impact of interpersonal violence trauma experiences and supporting the victim's/survivor's health and well-being outcomes. I believe that most of us who have chosen to work with people who engage in occupations that are 'in the shadows' are fierce advocates for social justice, not least because victims/survivors of trauma can be oppressed, shamed, silenced, and multiply marginalised. One must be motivated to do this difficult, emotion work. The double burden of the work itself and the consequent education and explanation to others can be daunting. The dark side of occupations is utilised as a framework to shape understanding and offers a useful approach to articulate the challenges of identifying and considering these individuals and the occupations they engage in, whether by choice or as victims/survivors.

My role in bringing interpersonal violence to the occupational therapy agenda

I began my work in the area of domestic violence as the onsite evaluator for the *Chicago Homeless Children's Head Start Evaluation* at Family Rescue, Inc. in Chicago, Illinois, USA. In that role I spent 20 hours per week conducting an ethnographic evaluation of a Head Start demonstration project that was housed within a Transitional Housing Program for women and their children who had sought emergency shelter services for domestic violence. I was simultaneously completing my doctoral work in public health and working as an adjunct faculty member in occupational therapy at the University of Illinois at Chicago. Through my observations at the site and subsequent dissertation interviews with mothers and staff members, I began to define a role for occupational therapy practitioners with this population (Helfrich, 2000). I recognised that the occupational and life skill needs of this population were immense; however, they were not documented anywhere. At that time, we knew little more than under-reported statistics from emergency room data and domestic violence shelters for women. The idea that men needed shelters was only beginning to emerge, but there were no bonafide shelters. The most progressive forms of refuge were safe houses sponsored primarily by social agencies for gay men which consisted of a confidential list of people who would take a man into their home for temporary protection. It is notable that the first shelter for LGBT adults (The Jazzie's Place Shelter) opened in San Francisco, California, USA, in 2015 (Childers, 2016), and the first registered domestic violence shelter for men opened in 2017 in Batesville, Arkansas, USA.

Family Rescue, Inc., founded in 1981 in Chicago, Illinois, is a comprehensive domestic violence agency for women and children that, as of this writing, includes (1) the Rosenthal Family Lodge Emergency Shelter, (2) the Ridgeland Apartments and Children's Program (which was the first Transitional Housing Program in the United States), (3) Court Advocacy Program, (4) Community Outreach Program, and (5) New Heights Apartments (which opened in 2017 with 54 units of transitional and scattered-site housing for women with or without children who are/were victims of domestic violence) (Family Rescue, 2025). In addition, the Community Outreach Program included a pilot programme for men who were abusers which was considered very controversial at the time. I had the privilege of completing domestic violence training and working with Family Rescue as an evaluator and researcher and eventually served as President of their Board of Directors. Although I knew how significant Family Rescue's work was in the United States when it was recognised by the White House, I just assumed that work in the United Kingdom with domestic violence was more progressive because the first domestic violence refuge in the world opened in Chiswick, a district of the London borough of Hounslow, Great Britain, in 1971. However, as you will discover in Kim Jones' chapter, occupational therapy has only recently joined the team of service providers in the United Kingdom.

In terms of understanding the functional implications of domestic violence and its impact on people as occupational beings, the literature did not exist. To most healthcare practitioners, this meant that the problem of domestic violence was not relevant to them. Despite legislation in some states in the United States that required healthcare providers to screen women for domestic violence, nobody wanted to take responsibility for doing so. I found that even emergency room personnel and gynaecologists did not think this was an important area of inquiry. Thus, when I presented the potential role for occupational therapy, I was consistently met with resistance. I learned to expect an attack after (or during) every presentation I gave on the topic, including job talks for faculty positions. Rather than give up on a topic I thought was critically important, I did what every good occupational therapist does when faced with a challenge: I analysed my audience and adapted my arguments. I focused on the physical safety and environmental risks related to interpersonal violence and used analogies such as how we would never do a home assessment and not consider the presence of area rugs or the absence of grab bars for an individual's safety. It was difficult for therapists to challenge this argument. Still, they argued it was beyond our scope of practice. Despite a gross lack of support from colleagues, I refused to give up. I developed fieldwork opportunities for students, documented the need and role of occupational therapy, and addressed the need to recognise the functional challenges whenever I was given the opportunity.

To the surprise of many of my colleagues, I obtained funding in 1999 from the US Department of Education, National Institute for Disabilities and Rehabilitation Research (NIDRR, now NIDILRR), to study the prevalence of health and disability issues among women seeking shelter services, which included a longitudinal qualitative study of a subset of women with disabilities (Helfrich, 1999–2003). Domestic violence was considered an *emerging disability* by NIDRR. To conduct this research, we needed to adapt the National Health Interview Survey – Disability Supplement (administered by the US Census Bureau) to capture data related to traumatic experiences (Helfrich et al., 2008). The data allowed me to demonstrate that victims/survivors of domestic violence had higher rates of both depression and anxiety than women in the general population of the United States. I translated those findings to describe how occupations were impacted, which was the foundation of my work with domestic violence across the lifespan.

About this book

In proposing this book, we were met with concerns about all that would be missing from this discussion. Reviewers cautioned that focusing on woman-to-woman rape would exclude the plethora of sexual and gender identities (as Bex addresses in Chapter 4), that our focus was too specific in the absence of a more general understanding of interpersonal violence, and that violence should be understood as gendered as the worldwide data reflects. We acknowledge that a larger, more comprehensive volume is needed and have plans to do that in the future; however, we also believe that occupational therapy practitioners must begin to grapple with illuminating these under-explored or discussed occupations in small doses first, to understand and begin to discuss these issues. While I first published work in this area in 2000, I have never addressed it from this perspective – that interpersonal violence is a part of most everyone's life in one way or another. This is not readily acknowledged, discussed, or shared with others. The reasons it is not discussed are likely similar to the reasons victims/survivors do not disclose. We lack an accessible vocabulary, and we are reluctant or lack the means of opportunity to include these aspects of ourselves as part of our identity. The chapters in this volume confront that reluctance by illuminating the humanity that co-exists within the horror that is interpersonal violence.

After nearly three decades of advocating for the role of occupational therapy with victims/survivors and perpetrators of interpersonal and sexual violence, there remain crucial reasons why occupational therapy practitioners should be challenged to respond to the needs of victimised people, including the following:

1) Our literature is limited on the issue of interpersonal violence, rape, and sexual assault.
2) The experiences of occupational therapy practitioners who do (knowingly) work with victims/survivors (regardless of setting) requires exploration.
3) Occupational therapists are not widely and visibly working in interpersonal violence, rape, and sexual assault services.
4) Many occupational therapy education/curriculum standards either do not specify a standard relating to any form of 'abuse', 'trauma', or 'violence' (see, e.g., Occupational Therapy Council of Australia Ltd, 2018; Royal College of Occupational Therapists, 2019) or simply state 'trauma' without clarification of which type (see 2023 Accreditation Council for Occupational Therapy Education [ACOTE®] Standards), despite the World Federation of Occupational Therapists' (WFOT) (2016) Minimum

Standards for the Education of Occupational Therapists doing so. In the latter named (WFOT) standards, they assert graduates need foundational

> Knowledge of theories and research findings about. . . . How to manage disruption to body structure or function to preserve the potential to participate in occupation . . . [including] Early childhood experiences of trauma, abuse and neglect with lifelong relational consequence.
>
> (2016, pp. 30–31)

However, many occupational therapy education/curriculum standards of WFOT-approved occupational therapy programmes do not specify any standard considerate of 'trauma', as discussed further in Chapter 5.

In this book, we analyse the limited exploration of interpersonal violence from an occupational perspective. Primarily, we have chosen to focus on adult victims/survivors in this book because of our collective experiences of predominantly working with adults and some older adults. Additionally, we acknowledge the absence of available literature regarding adult experiences. As the quote from WFOT (2016) above illustrates, the need to learn about early childhood experiences is acknowledged, yet adult experiences are not referred to. Necessarily and valuably, child abuse (childhood trauma or adverse childhood experiences [ACEs]) has been well documented over time in the occupational therapy literature (e.g. Coleman, 1975; Davidson, 1995; Cooper, 2000; Javed et al., 2020; Mazzeo & Bendixen, 2023), though it remains absent from most educational curriculum standards. This text does not specifically cover 'elder abuse', although there are older adults involved in some of the work described. Elder abuse is a complex phenomenon and is often covered under different legislation than interpersonal violence, which is beyond the scope of this book to address adequately (Atkinson & Roberto, 2024).

These facts bring us back to the need for this book. Despite the work that has been done, there is so much more to understand. The available data on interpersonal violence remains inaccurately low. This is due to a combination of the lack of agreed-upon understandings of what constitutes violence, lack of awareness of who the victims/survivors and perpetrators are, as well as the absence of robust data collection processes. WHO (2024b) currently reports that one in three women worldwide experience intimate partner violence during their lifetime; this historical trend in reporting intimate partner violence as an "overwhelming global burden . . . borne by women" (WHO, 2012) is, we would argue, flawed, given the focus in research and gathering of statistical prevalence data has involved women as data samples. While not to detract from the reality and gravity of women's experiences of violence perpetrated by men, all other victims/survivors and perpetrators need examining for a deeper understanding of the issues. Nobody is immune from this experience, while certain individuals are at greater risk, as will be discussed in this book.

Definitions are inconsistent within and between populations, services are inadequate, and methods for identification and documentation are woefully insufficient. The diversity of contexts and relationships in which interpersonal violence occurs among adults is endless. Interpersonal violence may be physical, sexual, or psychological and includes rape, sexual assault, intimate partner (dating or relationship) violence, and stalking. Acts of interpersonal violence are further divided into family or intimate partner violence (occurring within the family or between intimate partners) and community violence (occurring among individuals not related by family connections but who may or may not know each other). Globally, interpersonal violence is more than a pervasive public health problem; it is also a human right, economic, and development challenge (WHO, 2024b). In all its forms, the perpetration of interpersonal violence between adults cannot be denied, with the COVID-19 global pandemic highlighting and exacerbating its prevalence in our communities (WHO, 2020).

We have chosen to highlight three specific areas of interpersonal violence that have been absent from the literature: violence against women in the United Kingdom, woman-to-woman rape and sexual assault, and stalking behaviours. The author of each chapter will identify their positionality, present the identified issue using the framework of the dark side of occupation to illustrate the relevance to, and role of, occupational therapy, and present recommendations. The reader will notice there is intentional overlap between these chapters to emphasise the application to different populations. The final chapter synthesises the common threads and discusses areas of future work that are needed. However, each of us acknowledge that this text is a first for occupational therapy and for occupational science, and given the limitations of, for example, populations and the Global North geographical regions the work described covers, we end with appreciation of this and a hope for the generation of further contributions to this field of enquiry. This collection is intended to give practitioners, educators, students, and researchers manageable content to read and understand across a range of issues about interpersonal violence that are incorporated in this proposed text.

Defining terms and language used

Use of language is important when representing people's experiences, as Louis and the Sexual Violence Research Initiative assert: "Language and terms have been reclaimed by individuals and groups to ensure that their narratives are authentically voiced and portrayed appropriately" (2021, p. 2). There are several stylistic and vocabulary issues I will briefly discuss.

First, we, as authors, acknowledge this text is written in English and the use of any specific language introduces bias in terms of meanings and understanding communicated, in addition to considering the linguistic colonialism of English which therefore excludes or underrepresents certain individuals or groups.

Second, terminology varies when discussing domestic violence versus dating violence versus partner abuse versus intimate partner violence and victims versus survivors. As of 2018, the UK Home Office defines domestic violence and abuse as:

> Any incident or pattern of incidents of controlling, coercive, threatening behaviour, violence or abuse between those aged 16 or over who are, or have been, intimate partners or family members regardless of gender or sexual orientation. The abuse can encompass but is not limited to: psychological; physical; sexual; economic; emotional.
>
> (HM Government, 2018)

Terminology also varies geographically.

Third, legislations of any form of interpersonal violence vary globally. The three chapters by Kim, Sam, and Bex are all written in the context of UK (England and Wales) legislations, as is considered. Some countries, however, lack regulations as they do not have legislation or, instead, have unwritten laws for, for example, intimate partner (domestic) violence. Thus, we alert readers to become familiar with the language and laws pertaining to your location.

Fourth, we use the term victim(s)/survivor(s) for the following reasons. There has been extensive discussion regarding using the term victim versus survivor in both the grey and peer reviewed literature (e.g. Western et al., 2024; Women against Abuse, 2025). The discussions generally argue that 'victim' refers to someone who has experienced a crime and is experiencing trauma, while 'survivor' communicates empowerment and healing from trauma. There is an acknowledged necessity for the use of both terms which, within the Western criminal justice system, "have their place and serve different purposes. Although victim is a legal definition necessary within the criminal justice system, survivor can be used as a term of empowerment" (Sexual Assault Kit Initiative, n.d., p. 1). These terms are very meaningful to the individual to whom they refer, and both are used in a variety of settings and circumstances. Therefore, in most cases we use both as 'victim/survivor'. Additionally, as Twinley (2016, pp. 233–234) explained:

> After being victimised, survival takes multifarious forms, ranging from self-defence, managing past and recent traumatic experiences, and a determination to continue to live on – all of which are examples of the human capacity to survive. Hence my use of the term victim/survivor which, as Taylor (2004, p. 5) explains, describes:
>
> the reality of victimisation as well as the fact that the person who is victimised also survives – survives and conquers a crime that society is still unable to deal with effectively.

Finally, with an awareness that some languages (such as Persian and Chinese) either have a gender-neutral form or do not assign pronouns to a gender, it is important to us, as a writing team, to write "in a way that does not discriminate against a particular sex, social gender or gender identity, and does not perpetuate gender stereotypes" (UN, 2024). Though not without its limitations, we use gender-neutral and inclusive language, unless discussing the specifics (e.g. in terms of either sex or gender) of cases. In Chapter 4, Bex refers to the term 'trans' (as used by one of her respondents) which is used in the United Kingdom as a shorter form for 'transgender' and is used as "a general term for people whose gender is different from the gender assigned to them at birth" (Government Equalities Office, 2018, p. 1).

Interpersonal violence in all its forms (intimate partner violence, rape, and stalking) impacts all people, despite the common belief that men exclusively direct violence to women. Although the most commonly documented violence perpetrated by men is against women, often in intimate relationships, it is well documented that intimate partner violence occurs in all types of relationships (US Centers for Disease Control and Prevention, 2024). Unfortunately, the statistics for underrepresented groups are so much sparser than those for violence against women, as perpetrated by men.

Embracing our subjectivity

As you have already ascertained, this book is written in the first person. This approach is intentional to allow the authors to convey their stories in their own words. These are difficult topics to discuss, and we want the reader to experience the passion and respect conveyed in each chapter. As Letherby (who was Bex Twinley's Doctoral Studies Lead) explains: "Morley (1996) argues, when we use 'I' we question traditional styles of academic writing where 'we', 'the author' and 'he' are meant to represent distance and objectivity. 'I' is therefore a way of challenging traditional academic 'authority'" (2003, p. 7). Hence, rather than writing ourselves 'out' of our work, writing in the first person of 'I' essentially reflects how each of us has embraced our subjectivity and the significance of our personhood within our practice/research and writing. Letherby (2022, p. 16) helpfully explains the consequence of this choice:

> I suggest that, ironically, this acknowledgement of subjectivity and the associated 'super-sensitivity' to the relevance of the personhood of the researcher could feasibly lead to the conclusion that our work is more objective in that our work, although not value-free, is value-explicit.
>
> (Letherby, 2003, 2013)

Reading traumatic material

The authors each present an area where they have conducted foundational work in different areas of interpersonal violence. That work goes beyond academics. Nobody can do this work without a personal and emotional impact, as we discuss more in Chapter 5. In their respective chapters, the authors discuss the impact of working in these areas, as I have done in this introduction. This impact has compelled us to each consider our emotional safety. In each of our roles, being a disclosure recipient of interpersonal violence entails learning of traumatic and difficult events which, in turn, necessitates being aware of our own reactions to disclosures and managing our emotional reactions (Ullman, 2000). While this work is vital in the role of occupational therapy, we again caution that each reader must reflect on their response and take care to protect themselves, both emotionally and physically. As you read this book, we encourage you to pay attention to your own reactions and take breaks or seek support or supervision, as needed. We encourage you to acknowledge your own positionality and how this might influence your personal, emotional, and/or professional reactions. Think of your support network and those around you who understand the impact of these topics, be it a personal connection, a mentor, supervisor, or therapist/counsellor, and reach out for support.

What to consider as you read this book

As we have discussed, the material in this book may be sensitive or emotionally provocative or upsetting you as a reader. In addition, it may have an impact on you as a professional or student and/or as a victim/survivor yourself. We encourage you to consider the people you interact and work with. It is very likely that you do or will know people who are victims/survivors that you are not aware of.

References

Atkinson, E., & Roberto, K.A. (2024). Global approaches to primary, secondary, and tertiary elder abuse prevention: A scoping review. *Trauma, Violence, & Abuse*, *25*(1), 150–165.

Childers, L. (2016, May 31). *Nation's first LGBT adult homeless shelter opens in San Francisco*. https://www.calhealthreport.org/2016/05/31/nations-first-lgbt-adult-homeless-shelter-opens-in-san-francisco/

Coleman, W. (1975). Occupational-therapy and child abuse. *The American Journal of Occupational Therapy*, *29*(7), 412–417.

Cooper, R.J. (2000). The impact of child abuse on children's play: A conceptual model. *Occupational Therapy International*, *7*(4), 259–276. https://doi.org/10.1002/oti.127

Davidson, D.A. (1995). Physical abuse of preschoolers: Identification and intervention through occupational therapy. *The American Journal of Occupational Therapy*, *49*(3), 235–243. https://doi.org.ezproxy.brighton.ac.uk/10.5014/ajot.49.3.235

Family Rescue. (2025). *History of family rescue*. https://familyrescueinc.org/about/history-of-family-rescue/

Government Equalities Office. (2018). *Trans people in the UK*. Crown Copyright. https://assets.publishing.service.gov.uk/media/5b3a478240f0b64603fc181b/GEO-LGBT-factsheet.pdf

Helfrich, C.A. (2000). Domestic violence: Implications & guidelines for occupational therapy practitioners. In P. Rita & F. Cottrell (Eds.), *Proactive approaches in psychosocial occupational therapy* (pp. 309–316). Slack.

Helfrich, C.A. (Principal Investigator). (1999–2003). *A multi-level analysis of the relationship between domestic violence and disability*. U.S. Department of Education, National Institute on Disability and Rehabilitation Research, $449,476.

Helfrich, C.A., Fujiura, G., & Rutkowski, V. (2008). Mental health disorders and functioning of women in domestic violence shelters. *Journal of Interpersonal Violence*, *23*, 437–453. https://doi.org/10.1177/0886260507312942

HM Government. (2018, March 8). *Transforming the response to domestic abuse: Government consultation*, 13. https://publications.parliament.uk/pa/cm201719/cmselect/cmhaff/1015/101505.htm#footnote-162

Javed, U., Shawana, S., & Haroon, S. (2020). Role of occupational therapy on depression, anxiety and self-esteem of abused children. *Pakistan Journal of Rehabilitation*, *9*(2), 54–59. https://ojs.zu.edu.pk/pjr/article/view/997

Letherby, G. (2003). *Feminist research in theory and practice*. Open University Press.

Letherby, G. (2022). Thirty years and counting: An-other auto/biographical story. *Auto/Biography Review*, *3*(1), 13–31. https://doi.org/10.56740/abrev.v3i1.7

Louis, E.F., & Sexual Violence Research Initiative. (2021). *SVRI knowledge exchange: The power of language and its use in the GBV field*. SVRI. https://www.svri.org/sites/default/files/attachments/2021-11-25/SVRI_Knowledge_Exchange_Power_of_Language.pdf

Mazzeo, G., & Bendixen, R. (2023). Community-based interventions for childhood trauma: A scoping review. *OTJR: Occupational Therapy Journal of Research*, *43*(1), 14–23. https://doi.org/10.1177/15394492221091718

Njelesani, J., Tang, A., Jonsson, H., & Polatajko, H. (2014). Articulating an occupational perspective. *Journal of Occupational Science*, *21*(2), 226–235. https://doi.org/10.1080/14427591.2012.717500

Occupational Therapy Council of Australia Ltd. (2018). Accreditation Standards for Entry-Level Occupational Therapy Education Programs (December 2018). *Occupational Therapy Council of Australia Ltd.* https://www.otcouncil.com.au/wp-content/uploads/OTC-Accred-stds-and-criteria-December-2018-effective-January-2020.pdf

Royal College of Occupational Therapists (2019). The Learning and development standards for pre-registration education (Revised edition 2019). *Royal College of Occupational Therapists*. https://www.rcot.co.uk/practice-resources/rcot-publications/learning-and-development-standards-pre-registration-education

Sexual Assault Kit Initiative. (n.d.). *Victim or survivor: Terminology from investigation through prosecution*. https://sakitta.org/toolkit/docs/Victim-or-Survivor-Terminology-from-Investigation-Through-Prosecution.pdf

Twinley, R. (2016). *The perceived impacts of woman-to-woman rape and sexual assault, and the subsequent experience of disclosure, reaction, and support on victim/survivors' subjective experience of occupation.* [Doctoral dissertation, University of Plymouth] PEARL. https://pearl.plymouth.ac.uk/ handle/10026.1/6551

Twinley, R. (2021). The dark side of occupation: An introduction to the naming, creation, development, and intent of the concept. In R. Twinley (Ed.), *Illuminating the dark side of occupation: International perspectives from occupational therapy and occupational science* (1st ed., pp. 1–14). Routledge. https://doi.org/10.4324/9780429266256

Ullman, S.E. (2000). Psychometric characteristics of the social reactions questionnaire. *Psychology of Women Quarterly*, *24*(3), 257–271. https://doi.org/10.1111/j.1471-6402.2000.tb00208.x

United Nations (UN). (2024). *Gender-inclusive language*. https://www.un.org/en/gender-inclusive-language/

US Centers for Disease Control and Prevention. (2024, May 16). *About intimate partner violence*. https://www.cdc.gov/intimate-partner-violence/about/index.html

Western, K.A.B., Cruwys, T., & Evans, O. (2024). Identifying as a survivor versus a victim after sexual violence predicts divergent posttrauma pathways. *Violence against Women*, *0*(0). https://doi.org/10.1177/10778012241279817

Women against Abuse. (2025). *The language we use*. https://www.womenagainstabuse.org/education-resources/the-language-we-use

World Federation of Occupational Therapists (WFOT) (2016). Minimum Standards for the Education of Occupational Therapists. *World Federation of Occupational Therapists*. https://wfot.org/resources/new-minimum-standards-for-the-education-of-occupational-therapists-2016-e-copy

World Health Organization (WHO). (2012). *Understanding and addressing violence against women: Intimate partner violence*. https://apps.who.int/iris/bitstream/handle/10665/77432/WHO_RHR_12.36_eng.pdf

World Health Organization (WHO). (2020, April 7). *COVID-19 and violence against women*. https://iris.who.int/bitstream/handle/10665/331699/WHO-SRH-20.04-eng.pdf?sequence=1

World Health Organization (WHO). (2024a). *The VPA (Violence Prevention Alliance) approach*. https://www.who.int/groups/violence-prevention-alliance/approach

World Health Organization (WHO). (2024b, March 13). *Violence against women*. https://www.who.int/news-room/fact-sheets/detail/violence-against-women

2 Intimate partner violence

Rebuilding occupational identity using occupational therapy

Kim Jones

Background and positionality

To contextualise this work and address potential bias, I reflect on my extensive experience in the field of intimate partner violence, spanning over 15 years. In this role, I provided both practical and emotional support to victims/survivors, including devising safety plans and facilitating access to essential services. Despite these efforts, I observed a recurring pattern: even after achieving physical separation and receiving external support, many individuals continued to struggle with the psychological and emotional grip of their experiences.

Motivated to address these deeper needs, I qualified as a counsellor to help individuals express and process their emotions. While this approach offered temporary relief, I sought more sustainable methods to facilitate recovery. My discovery of occupational therapy provided the holistic framework I was searching for, empowering survivors to rebuild essential aspects of their lives and fostering lasting transformation.

During a role-emerging occupational therapy placement, I witnessed first-hand the transformative potential of this approach. Observing victims/survivors rediscover meaningful and purposeful occupational identities profoundly shaped my commitment to innovation and advocacy in this field, ultimately defining the trajectory of my professional journey (Jones, 2020). In this chapter, I will illuminate how I learnt intimate partner violence was found to affect a person's social and cognitive function, and – from an occupational perspective – I uncover the less understood impacts on victims'/survivors' occupational lives, including their daily living skills, the ability to carry out valued roles, the management of interpersonal relationships, and their ability to engage in employment.

Overview of intimate partner violence

Intimate partner violence (also referred to as dating or relationship violence) refers to abuse occurring between individuals who are 'per

DOI: 10.4324/9781032726878-2

sonally connected'. This connection includes relationships such as the following:

- Married or civil partnership couples (current or former).
- Those engaged to marry or enter a civil partnership.
- Individuals in an intimate personal relationship.
- Parents sharing a parental relationship for the same child.

Intimate partner violence encompasses behaviours such as coercive control, physical and sexual violence, threats, economic abuse, and psychological or emotional harm (U.S. Centers for Disease Control and Prevention, 2024).

Once an individual becomes part of an intimate partnership, they may find themselves trapped within the 'Cycle of Violence' (Walker, 1979). This recurring pattern, which can vary in duration from hours to months, includes phases of tension-building, abuse, and reconciliation, perpetuating a sense of entrapment. Figure 2.1 illustrates this dynamic, emphasising its non-linear and repetitive nature. The 'Cycle of Violence' typically involves four phases:

1. **Tension** – A stage characterised by an overwhelming mix of emotions, including humiliation, fear, hopelessness, and depression, which progressively hinder participation in daily activities.
2. **Incident** – An abusive event occurs, which may involve physical, emotional, or psychological harm where individuals may attempt to leave the relationship, though it typically takes up to seven attempts to achieve permanent separation.
3. **Reconciliation** – The abuser attempts to regain control, employing tactics such as gaslighting, excuses, or apologies, which create a false sense of reassurance.
4. **Calm or 'Honeymoon'** – The perpetrator promises that the abuse will not happen again, often accompanied by denial, blame-shifting, or declarations such as 'It was your fault' or 'I did it because I love you'.

Introduction to the project

This chapter presents an initiative aimed at delivering direct occupational therapy to individuals who have experienced Intimate Partner Violence, known as the 'Intimate Partner Violence and Occupational Therapy Project'. Conceptualised, developed, and implemented by myself in collaboration with Lucy Clarke, whose experience spans 33 years in the field of occupational therapy (Clarke & Jones, 2021), this project addressed the significant impacts of intimate partner violence on both the physical and emotional aspects of daily functioning.

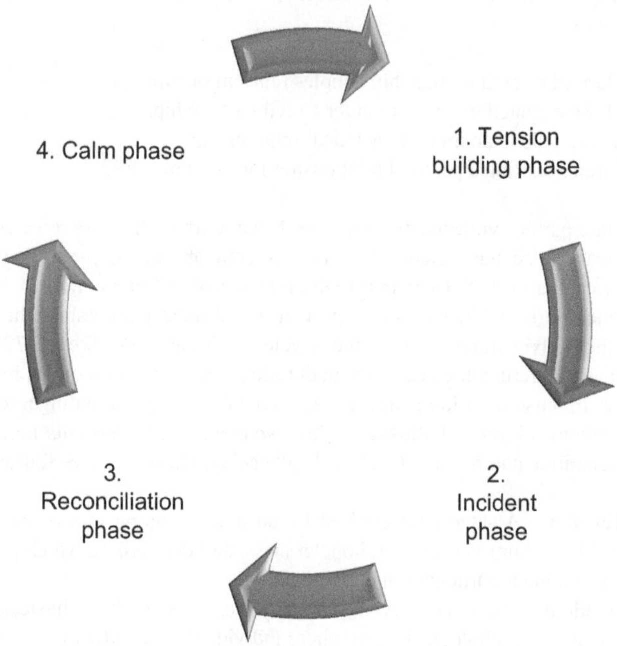

Figure 2.1 Illustration of the cycle of violence

Intimate partner violence specifically refers to harmful behaviours – ranging from physical, emotional, and psychological to sexual abuse – within romantic or intimate relationships, regardless of cohabitation or marital status. This is distinct from the broader concept of 'domestic abuse/violence', which encompasses abuse within family settings, involving various household members, children, or cohabitants (Women against Abuse, 2025). This chapter focuses on intimate partner violence within the context of dating and romantic relationships, with particular attention to the unique dynamics and challenges they present.

Recognising these complexities, the project sought to address the specific needs of victim-survivors through a holistic, evidence-based occupational therapy approach. By leveraging the principles of The Model of Human Occupation (Taylor et al., 2023), the aim was to empower individuals to rebuild their lives, regain independence, and reclaim their sense of identity through meaningful engagement in daily occupations.

Defining the role of occupational therapy

Historically, the role of occupational therapy in supporting intimate partner violence victims/survivors has been underdefined. However, work completed by Helfrich and Aviles (Helfrich, 2001) supported the development of this project by providing a framework for understanding the impact of domestic abuse on occupational performance and participation. In *Domestic Abuse Across the Lifespan: The Role of Occupational Therapy*, Helfrich (2001) emphasises the critical importance of trauma-informed interventions tailored to survivors' needs. Her exploration of a lifespan approach highlighted how abuse disrupts routines, roles, and engagement in meaningful activities, directly informing the design of interventions used in the pilot I was involved in.

For example, Helfrich's focus on rebuilding self-esteem and fostering independence influenced the adoption of tools such as the Canadian Occupational Performance Measure (COPM) to assess progress. Additionally, her work on multi-agency collaboration underscored the importance of engaging with a broad network of professionals, a strategy that became central to our project's success. Moreover, drawing on over 15 years of experience in the intimate partner violence field and my professional expertise as an occupational therapist, I developed and evaluated the Domestic Abuse Occupational Therapy Project in North Wales (Clarke & Jones, 2021). This project marked a significant milestone in clarifying and advancing the role of occupational therapy in addressing the complex needs of intimate partner violence survivors, integrating both theoretical foundations and practical innovation.

Foundations for developing the project: insights and knowledge

The project sought to establish an occupational therapy service offering early intervention and mental health rehabilitation 'upstream'. The aim was to embed self-management strategies into survivors' daily routines, enabling recovery from the trauma of domestic abuse. Guided by a person-centred approach, the service focused on the following:

- Identifying individually meaningful occupational goals for daily living post-abuse.
- Supporting the development of occupational identity through meaningful activities and roles in home, family, and community life.

Additionally, the project leveraged a network of health, social care, and third-sector providers to deliver prudent and effective support to individuals seeking assistance.

The project's implementation coincided with the COVID-19 lockdown, a period that exacerbated stress responses and heightened the frequency and severity of intimate partner violence incidents (Office for National Statistics, 2020). Lockdown conditions created challenges in service delivery, including limited access to one-on-one appointments and virtual support. Survivors faced significant barriers to privacy and digital access, and the suspension of community activities further isolated them.

Occupational therapy played a critical role in addressing these challenges. Through holistic interventions, occupational therapy helped survivors rebuild their identities and regain independence. The integration of academic knowledge, professional frameworks, and personal expertise laid a robust foundation for understanding the occupational and social impacts of intimate partner violence.

The economic cost of intimate partner violence in England and Wales is estimated at £66 billion annually, equating to over £34,000 per person affected (Oliver et al., 2019). This figure encompasses costs related to lost work time, professional support services, hospital visits, housing support, and social service interventions for both adults and children. The Equality and Human Rights Commission (n.d.) state: "In the UK, in any one year, more than 20% of employed women take time off work because of domestic violence, and 2% lose their jobs as a direct result of the abuse".

Through this project, we gained deeper insights into the pervasive nature of intimate partner violence, which transcends demographics and profoundly impacts individuals' physical, emotional, and occupational well-being. The research further illuminated the dynamics of coercive control (Monckton-Smith, 2023) and the Cycle of Violence (Walker, 1979), providing critical context for addressing the needs of survivors.

Examining outcomes and empowering victims/survivors

Through an analysis of outcome measures, this project explored how intimate partner violence affects social and cognitive functioning from an occupational perspective. Beyond the well-documented physical and emotional effects, I examined the disruptions intimate partner violence causes to daily living skills, challenges in fulfilling meaningful roles, difficulties managing interpersonal relationships, and barriers to employment (Law et al., 2014; Fuller, 2011).

Occupational therapy interventions enabled victims/survivors to work collaboratively with their families and communities, fostering the development of their occupational identity. This process facilitated the mastery of new or enhanced roles and routines, contributing to a more meaningful and empowered occupational life (Kielhofner, 2008).

The occupational therapy initiative: a holistic approach to victim/survivor support

This project was implemented within a community setting in collaboration with a local charitable organisation, aiming to address the multifaceted needs of victims/survivors of intimate partner violence.

Background

The heightened incidence of intimate partner violence following the COVID-19 pandemic posed significant challenges to the physical and emotional well-being of victims/survivors. This increase negatively impacted their daily lives, affecting their occupational lives in terms of their social and cognitive functioning, interpersonal relationships, employment, and daily living skills.

Challenges

The establishment of this new service faced unique hurdles due to the ongoing lockdown measures implemented during COVID-19. Victims/survivors often had to prioritise home-schooling responsibilities and struggled to attend one-on-one appointments. Access to virtual support services was inconsistent, as privacy and access to digital technology were not universally available. Furthermore, many community activities, support services, and third-sector programmes remained closed or operated with limited virtual offerings, leaving survivors further isolated.

These constraints also limited opportunities for group work, which could not be safely offered during this period. Networking with partner organisations had to be conducted remotely or in small, socially distanced groups. Over the course of the project, it became clear that employing additional occupational therapy assistant practitioners would enhance the service's efficiency. These practitioners would support the practical application of skills developed during therapy, furthering the initiative's reach and impact.

Key interventions and outcomes

To initiate the project, approximately 500 professionals from partner organisations with a connection to domestic abuse were contacted, educated, and influenced. This was achieved through a combination of emails, face-to-face interactions, and Teams meetings. Feedback from multidisciplinary and multi-agency colleagues highlighted the positive impact of the occupational therapist on team morale, victim/survivor engagement, and multi-agency collaboration. Comprehensive documents and processes were developed to establish an occupational therapy pathway from referral through to discharge, which are now prepared for broader adoption across Wales.

During the nine-month pilot phase, I engaged with 30 women aged 18 and over. Of these, 20 actively participated in occupational therapy interventions, with 15 demonstrating significant improvements in their ability to perform chosen occupations, as measured by the COPM (Law et al., 2019). One participant chose not to complete the outcome measures. Additionally, eight onward referrals were made to address significant risks identified during the project. To provide a clearer understanding of the specific interventions utilised during the project, Table 2.1 outlines the key occupational therapy interventions.

Having outlined the key personal goals identified across participants in Table 2.1, I will examine the contents further and provide an in-depth discussion of the interventions used to address each goal. I include how I developed my practice and tailored intervention to meet the unique needs of victims/survivors, as individuals, along with the challenges faced in delivering these interventions. Through this detailed analysis, I aim to highlight the practical application of occupational therapy techniques in supporting victims'/survivors' recovery and the restoration of their occupational identities, discussing key challenges encountered.

Anxiety management

Intervention

In working with survivors of intimate partner violence, managing anxiety was frequently identified as a primary goal. I employed cognitive-behavioural therapy (CBT) approach, mindfulness practices, and relaxation strategies to help individuals manage their anxiety, ultimately enabling them to engage more effectively in their chosen occupations and goals. Through these interventions, I empowered the individual to identify anxiety triggers, regulate emotional responses, and develop personalised coping mechanisms that could be utilised in various life situations.

Table 2.1 Occupational therapy interventions related to participant goals

Personal goals identified in COPMs across the participants	*Number of times goals identified across the cohort*	*Categories*
1) Manage Anxiety	10	Symptom Management
2) Activities of Daily Living (ADLs)	9	Self-Care
3) Attend College/University	8	Roles
4) Meaningful Activities	7	Leisure
5) Social Contact	6	Sense of Belonging
6) Maintaining Home	6	Roles
7) Attend/Maintain/Return Work	5	Roles
8) Sleep Hygiene	5	Establish Routine
9) Develop Structure	5	Establish Routine
10) Parenting	4	Roles
11) Manage Low Mood	4	Symptom Management
12) Pain Management	2	Symptom Management
13) Exercise	2	Self-Care
14) Pacing Activity	1	Symptom Management

Psychoeducation on anxiety and emotional regulation played a central role in the process, helping survivors understand how anxiety manifests and how it affected their daily functioning. By integrating practical strategies like controlled breathing, grounding exercises, and progressive muscle relaxation, I supported the development of skills that allowed individuals to remain grounded and regain control in moments of distress.

Challenges

Anxiety often emerges as part of a broader trauma response and can significantly hinder an individual's ability to function in daily life. Survivors struggled with feelings of heightened vulnerability, fear, and difficulty in trusting others. These emotional barriers made engagement in therapeutic activities particularly challenging. As a result, our interventions were tailored to each survivor's pace. In many cases, therapy began with shorter, manageable sessions to foster a sense of safety and build rapport. Ensuring that the victim/survivor felt supported and understood while creating a therapeutic environment. Through consistent, empathetic engagement, I was able to guide the victim/survivor in gradually confronting and managing their anxiety within the context of their broader recovery process.

Activities of daily living

Intervention

In working with victims/survivors of intimate partner violence, a key focus was on restoring their ability to perform their everyday occupations (termed in the service as 'ADLs') without fear, particularly self-care tasks, such as personal hygiene, grooming, dressing, and feeding. These activities are often significantly disrupted due to the trauma, fear, and disempowerment victims/survivors experience. My role was to assess each individual's unique challenges and abilities, then provide tailored support aimed at re-establishing routines that facilitated these essential activities.

To address these challenges, I implemented strategies such as structuring daily routines, creating visual schedules, and incorporating adaptive equipment where necessary. For instance, visual reminders helped individuals plan and sequence their self-care tasks, while adaptive tools ensured that tasks like dressing or grooming were more manageable and less overwhelming. The overall goal was to empower individuals by helping them regain a sense of control and independence in these basic activities, thereby fostering a sense of self-worth and normality.

Challenge

A significant challenge in supporting the intimate partner violence survivors in maintaining personal care was the pervasive impact of anxiety, trauma, and a lack of self-worth. These emotional and psychological barriers often led to neglect of self-care routines, with survivors feeling disconnected from their own bodies and identities. I felt it was crucial to approach these barriers with sensitivity, understanding the deep emotional and cognitive effects of the trauma survivors had experienced. Interventions needed to be gradual and empowerment-focused, emphasising the survivor's capacity to regain confidence and control over their own care. This process required patience and a strong therapeutic relationship built on trust, enabling survivors to work towards reclaiming their personal care routines without feeling overwhelmed or judged.

Attending college/university

Intervention

Returning to education was a powerful step for many of our survivors in rebuilding their lives and sense of identity. I designed interventions to support them to re-engage with educational goals, such as attending college or university. These interventions focused on helping individuals develop effective study routines, manage time, and address cognitive challenges linked to trauma, such as difficulty with concentration and memory. To assist with these challenges, we often broke down academic tasks into smaller, more manageable steps, utilising assistive technology and creating an optimal environment conducive to learning. This structured approach supported survivors in regaining confidence in their intellectual abilities, empowering them to succeed in their educational pursuits.

Challenge

For many of our survivors, returning to education was daunting due to emotional and cognitive barriers. Previous experiences of failure or trauma had left them feeling inadequate or fearful of judgement in an academic setting. Overcoming these barriers requires a patient, trauma-informed approach where survivors are supported not only in building academic skills but also in addressing any lingering emotional and cognitive obstacles that may hinder their participation.

Meaningful activities

Intervention

Engaging in meaningful (including leisure) activities played a critical role in helping the victims/survivors we worked with reconnect with themselves and, even, rediscover a sense of joy. As part of our interventions, I assisted individuals in identifying leisure activities that resonate with their interests and promote relaxation, enjoyment, and social connection. Examples include engaging in hobbies such as painting, gardening, or reading, or participating in group sports or crafts. These activities are not only therapeutic but also help individuals rebuild their sense of identity beyond the trauma they have experienced, reinforcing a positive self-image and a healthy balance of life.

Challenge

Re-engaging in leisure activities was found challenging due to emotional barriers which brought them joy, which was often difficult for them to prioritise activities outside of survival. We worked gradually, reintroducing activities in a way that was manageable and supportive of their emotional state. We often focused on overcoming emotional barriers, addressing issues of self-worth, and fostering social engagement to support this.

Social contact

Intervention

Social isolation was again a significant issue for many of the victims/survivors. My work played a crucial role in helping individuals rebuild their social networks by identifying safe, supportive environments and fostering effective communication skills. Additionally, we included facilitating group activities, discussion of social and interpersonal communication and interaction skills, and encouraged community involvement. By providing these opportunities, I was able to help victims/survivors regain their confidence in social settings, rebuild trust, and cultivate a sense of belonging and connection.

Challenge

Due to past abuse, survivors struggled with distrust or fear in social situations. The trauma they have experienced made it difficult for them to feel comfortable in group settings or even in one-on-one interactions. Our interventions focused on increasing social engagement in a graduated manner, often starting with one-on-one meetings or small group activities in safe, non-judgemental spaces. This allowed survivors to rebuild social skills, restore their sense of self-worth, and gain confidence in their ability to interact with others.

Maintaining home

Intervention

Maintaining a home environment was a key role for the victims/survivors attending the project, due to it providing a sense of stability and control.

I worked with individuals to develop strategies for organising household tasks, managing finances, and ensuring that the living environment was safe and comfortable. This involved creating structured routines for meal planning, scheduling household chores, or implementing environmental modifications to make the space more functional. These interventions supported survivors in reclaiming their role within the home, promoting independence and a sense of accomplishment.

Challenge

For many victims/survivors, the effects of trauma lead to fatigue, confusion, or an inability to focus, to complete household management. We often had to break tasks down into smaller, manageable steps and use adaptive tools to help them engage in home management tasks. Additionally, addressing issues such as organisational support or financial assistance was also necessary for victims/survivors.

Attend/maintain/return to work

Intervention

Within this area I supported by addressing the physical, emotional, and cognitive barriers that arose. This involved helping survivors explore suitable work roles, manage time, and navigate workplace accommodations. Also, the interventions included addressing workplace dynamics to ensure they felt supported in their return to work. These strategies were designed to foster work readiness and enable survivors to rebuild their professional identity with confidence.

Challenge

The survivors experienced challenges related to self-confidence, fear of re-victimisation, and trauma-related cognitive difficulties (e.g. trouble concentrating). Returning to work required overcoming these barriers and identifying strategies that enable them to thrive in a professional environment. Additionally, together we included setting realistic goals and provided emotional support through the process.

Sleep hygiene

Intervention

Many of the survivors experienced significant sleep disturbances, including nightmares and insomnia, as a result of trauma. Interventions focused on establishing consistent sleep routines, creating a calming sleep environment, and introducing relaxation techniques to improve sleep quality. This included strategies like progressive muscle relaxation, deep breathing, or guided imagery to help manage stress and encourage restorative sleep.

Challenge

Trauma-related sleep disturbances are complex; I was required to provide a tailored approach to each individual's needs. Working collaboratively with survivors to identify specific sleep barriers – whether psychological, physical, or environmental – and develop a routine that addressed their issues. This process required patience, as sleep hygiene often required adjustments to both psychological and physical aspects of the survivor's routine.

Develop structure

Intervention

Another key intervention was supporting survivors to develop structured routines that promoted stability and a sense of control. I assisted in creating daily schedules that prioritised self-care, meal planning, and leisure activities, all designed to bring structure and predictability to their daily life. This significantly improved the survivor's sense of autonomy and reduced feelings of chaos or helplessness.

Challenge

Trauma severely disrupted daily functioning, making it difficult for survivors to establish consistent routines. I was able to work flexibly and incrementally to support this. In many cases the goal was to empower the victim/survivor to regain control over their daily life while also being sensitive to the emotional toll of the recovery process.

Case study: an example of occupational therapy with a victim/survivor

To further illuminate the types of experiences for victims/survivors of intimate partner violence, the following case study illustrates its impact on a person's occupations of daily life.

Background

Mair,[1] a 27-year-old female, had endured a seven-year abusive relationship. Living alone, she found companionship and solace in caring for her dog and horse, which played a significant role in her emotional recovery and daily routine. Despite an attempt to leave the relationship two years earlier, Mair often experienced depression, anxiety, and suicidal ideations with reduced occupational identity. These challenges led her to return to the perpetrator, perceiving him as a source of safety and familiarity. This cycle of leaving and returning had repeated numerous times.

Since the end of the relationship, Mair faced significant barriers in her daily life, including difficulties maintaining her job, managing her home, and engaging in basic daily tasks. Although she had supportive family, friends, and colleagues, Mair's experiences had isolated her, leaving her feeling disconnected and without a sense of belonging.

Brief summary of assessments and interventions

Guided by a holistic occupational therapy approach, we developed tailored strategies to empower Mair to rebuild her routines, enhance her self-efficacy, and support her recovery journey.

The Occupational Circumstances Assessment Interview and Rating Scale (OCAIRS) (Forsyth & Model of Human Occupation Clearinghouse, 2006) was used to build a therapeutic relationship, identify Mair's strengths and values, and establish a foundation for a personalised intervention plan (Dixon & Roberts, 2013; Social Care Institute for Excellence, 2022). To monitor her mental health, the Patient Health Questionnaire-9 (PHQ-9) (Kroenke & Spitzer, 2002) and the Generalized Anxiety Disorder-7 Scale (Löwe et al., 2008) were employed, assessing levels of depression, anxiety, and suicidal ideations.

We completed a Role Checklist to help Mair identify, develop, and rebuild her values and roles (Scott et al., 2017). Additionally, the COPM (Law et al., 2014) was used to identify and prioritise meaningful goals for intervention, providing insight into her self-perception of occupational performance and satisfaction.

Interventions were designed to address Mair's mental health, daily functioning, and sense of purpose through evidence-based approaches.

Mair's journey began with addressing her mental health challenges, including anxiety and depression. Together, we discussed seeking additional support from her GP while integrating educational sessions to manage these concerns. These sessions explored practical strategies for anxiety and depression management, mindfulness practices, and sleep hygiene to promote overall well-being (Critcher & Dunning, 2015; Ingram & Luxton, 2005; Randal et al., 2015; Faulkner, 2017; Bothelius et al., 2013).

Through collaborative discussions, we set SMART goals, breaking down complex tasks into achievable steps and celebrating milestones to maintain momentum (Bovend'Eerdt et al., 2009). Using tools like the Role Checklist Version 3 (Scott et al., 2017) and incorporating the Five Ways to Wellbeing framework (Aked et al., 2008), we identified areas for growth and areas requiring support in Mair's occupational roles and routines. We developed strategies to establish positive routines that supported her work-life balance and home environment (Fritz & Cutchin, 2016). As Mair began to rebuild her roles and reconnect with meaningful activities, we used motivational interviewing techniques to help her explore new perspectives, boosting her confidence and commitment to change (Rollnick et al., 2008).

This tailored, multifaceted approach enabled Mair to regain a sense of control over her life, build resilience, and re-establish her occupational and personal identity (Mattingly & Lewandowski, 2013).

Number of contacts

Mair engaged in a total of nine sessions, delivered through a combination of phone consultations and socially distanced, face-to-face interactions.

Outcomes

All of Mair's selected goals, as identified and documented through the COPM, demonstrated measurable improvement. Outcome scores increased by two or more points across all goal areas in both performance and satisfaction domains (Law et al., 2014). Mair exhibited enhanced motivation, successfully maintaining her home and dedicating quality time to caring for her animals. Additionally, her sleep pattern improved, achieving a healthy and consistent range.

Mair also demonstrated sustained positive work habits, eliminating the risk of job loss. Furthermore, she re-established and maintained meaningful social connections, including friendships and family relationships, which contributed to her overall sense of well-being and belonging (Wilcock, 2002).

Client feedback

- 'I have enough tools to take forward, and build my new life'.
- 'I feel like my old self again'.
- 'Work have seen a massive change in my productivity, quality and concentration'.
- 'Spending time with my animals is more of a joy than a hindrance'.

Insights gained: implications and things to consider as occupational therapists

This initiative has shown the transformative potential of occupational therapy in addressing the complex needs of victims/survivors of intimate partner violence (domestic abuse). By equipping individuals with the skills and resources necessary to rebuild their lives, this pilot project has laid the groundwork for an innovative, scalable model of support across Wales.

Before initiating the project, we acknowledged that victims and survivors often become entrapped in the 'cycle of violence', characterised by a repetitive pattern of tension-building, incident, and reconciliation or calm phases, as outlined by Walker (1979). This cyclical dynamic underscores the profound psychological grip that abusive relationships exert on individuals. Observations revealed that while interventions such as medication, anxiety management, and practical support offer temporary relief, they frequently fall short in addressing the deeper challenge of rebuilding occupational identity.

Encouragingly, both quantitative and qualitative data collected during the project demonstrated how occupational therapy effectively supported survivors in establishing future goals, roles, routines, and structures, fostering long-term recovery and growth. However, our work also uncovered four key themes that illuminated hidden barriers, explaining why individuals often struggle to move beyond their traumatic past and fully engage in meaningful occupations.

As integral members of the multidisciplinary team, occupational therapists are uniquely positioned to address the immediate emotions and thoughts of victims/survivors, bridging the gap between present needs and future aspirations. These findings emphasise the complexity of the recovery process and the essential role of tailored, holistic interventions in overcoming these to rebuild their lives.

Identifying themes that illuminate hidden barriers

The process of identifying the themes of fear, love, grief, and vulnerability in the context of intimate partner violence was developed over a 12-year period as lead practitioner in domestic violence and child protection. During this time, patterns emerged from assessments and interventions with victims/survivors of intimate partner violence. By analysing responses to these assessments and observing how individuals engaged with various therapeutic interventions, certain recurring emotional and psychological themes became evident. These themes consistently appeared as central to the survivors' experiences, providing a framework through which to understand and address the profound impacts of intimate partner violence on their lives. The identification of these themes was not only informed by clinical observations but also supported by extensive research and theory, as evidenced by the work of key scholars in the field (Brown, 2015; Edhammer et al., 2024; Heron et al., 2022; Monckton-Smith, 2023).

Once I began my training as an occupational therapist, I was able to further connect this data to the field of occupational therapy and explore how recovery could be linked to meaningful occupations after a victim/survivor had left the abusive relationship. This deeper understanding allowed me to provide the missing piece in healing – the development of occupational identity (Hansson, 2021). By focusing on rebuilding the victims'/survivors' engagement in daily activities and routines that hold personal meaning, we were able to help victims/survivors regain a sense of autonomy, purpose, and well-being in the aftermath of intimate partner violence. Within this project the occupational therapy process became a vital part of their recovery, supporting not just physical and emotional healing but also the restoration of self-worth and identity.

Theme one: fear

Under this key theme, we identified two subthemes that represented the experience of fear: immediate fear and chronic fear.

Immediate fear

Immediate fear, triggered by acute threat, involves fight-or-flight reactions and emotional symptoms like panic or anger, with the primary focus on preserving safety in the moment (Monckton-Smith, 2023). In occupational therapy, this fear is addressed by helping individuals feel safe and supported, guiding them through immediate interventions such as developing coping mechanisms and crisis management strategies. By providing structured support during these heightened moments, occupational therapists enable survivors to regain a sense of control and security, laying the groundwork for longer-term healing and recovery.

Chronic fear

Chronic fear, developed over time in abusive environments, leads victims/survivors to adopt strategies like managing the abuser's behaviour and constantly assessing risks (Monckton-Smith, 2023). These adaptations focus more on anticipating harm than immediate danger, creating a state of insecurity. Occupational therapy plays a crucial role in addressing chronic fear by helping individuals regain a sense of control. Therapists work with survivors to develop coping strategies, restore routine, and rebuild occupational identity, ultimately empowering them to heal, establish safety, and disrupt the cycle of violence.

Theme two: love

Research highlights that love can be a compelling reason for victims/survivors to stay in abusive relationships, often making their situation even more challenging. This emotion can provoke deeply conflicting feelings, as individuals grapple with questions like, *'How can I love someone who hurts me?'* or *'What will people think if I admit that I still love them?'* It is essential to recognise that victims/survivors often experience the Cycle of Violence repeatedly – tension builds, an incident occurs, and then reconciliation, often accompanied by declarations of love, follows. This cycle reinforces emotional bonds and complicates the decision to leave (Heron et al., 2022).

Occupational therapy can support individuals navigating the complexities of love and attachment in abusive relationships by addressing the emotional, psychological, and occupational impacts from the Cycle of Violence. Through a trauma-informed approach, occupational therapists facilitate survivors' understanding of their experiences, providing a safe space to explore conflicting feelings and emotional bonds. This includes identifying how the cycle affects daily routines, roles, and self-perception. By collaboratively setting goals and focusing on meaningful occupations, therapy empowers victims/survivors to rebuild their occupational identity, develop healthy coping strategies, and regain a sense of autonomy and purpose.

Theme three: grief

Based on data collated during the project, survivors of intimate partner violence demonstrated profound grief associated with the loss of identity, safety, and roles integral to their daily lives. Occupational therapy interventions were crucial in addressing these disruptions by fostering adaptive coping mechanisms, rebuilding routines, and redefining meaningful roles. Through collaborative goal setting, therapeutic activities, and psychoeducation, survivors were supported to process grief, regain autonomy, and establish sustainable occupational identities, promoting long-term recovery and resilience in the wake of intimate partner violence.

Theme four: vulnerability

Vulnerability is a significant emotional response for victims of intimate partner violence, as they endure uncertainty, fear, and emotional exposure. Research by Brene Brown (2017) highlights that this vulnerability can manifest as anxiety, self-blame, and a desire to protect oneself, often causing victims to withdraw or lash out. Vulnerability places victims/survivors at a significantly increased risk of being re-victimised (Edhammer et al., 2024). For those experiencing intimate partner violence, this heightened state of vulnerability interferes with their ability to engage in meaningful activities and roles. Occupational therapists can play a crucial role in helping survivors by providing a supportive space, helping them rebuild self-worth, and addressing their emotional responses through therapeutic interventions.

Illuminating the dark side of occupation to understand impact

Early findings from this project highlighted the substantial variability in how individuals experience and respond to the trauma associated with intimate partner violence. Factors such as stress responses, age, and the frequency and severity of abuse significantly influenced these impacts. The power-control dynamics, characteristic of abusive relationships, played a pivotal role in shaping how victims/survivors engaged with their occupations, often limiting access to meaningful or essential activities and occupations while imposing restrictive roles or tasks.

The concept of the *dark side of occupations*, as explored from varying perspectives in *Illuminating the Dark Side of Occupation* (Twinley, 2021), provided a transformative lens to examine the lived experiences of victims/survivors, offering critical insights into how intimate partner violence profoundly disrupts daily life and overall well-being. This perspective illuminated the complex interplay between trauma and occupational engagement, highlighting how victims/survivors' participation in meaningful activities is often constrained or shaped by the abusive context. Twinley's work deepened my understanding of how coercion, control, and survival mechanisms influence occupational choices, laying a crucial foundation for developing trauma-informed, person-centred intervention strategies that support survivors in reclaiming their occupational identity and agency.

Conclusion

The Domestic Abuse Occupational Therapy Project stands as one of the most significant and impactful milestones of my professional journey. Observing survivors progress from vulnerability to empowerment reinforced my conviction in the transformative potential of occupational therapy. This initiative not only equipped survivors with practical tools and strategies to rebuild their lives but also contributed to the restoration of their confidence and sense of self. The positive outcomes surpassed our expectations, underscoring both the resilience of survivors and the critical importance of person-centred, trauma-informed care in facilitating meaningful recovery.

I am profoundly inspired by the resilience and determination demonstrated by the individuals we supported, and I take great pride in the role occupational therapy played in facilitating their journeys towards independence and recovery. This project has strengthened my commitment to advancing the profession's contributions to addressing Intimate Partner Violence and promoting meaningful, sustainable change in the lives of those impacted. It is my hope that this work will serve as a foundation for future innovation and inspire others to recognise and harness the transformative potential of occupational therapy in supporting individuals affected by intimate partner violence.

Future directions and recommendations

Future research should build upon the findings of this project by extending its scope to explore the occupational and psychological impacts of intimate partner violence across diverse populations. Pursuing a PhD would facilitate a more in-depth examination of how intimate partner violence disrupts occupational identity and function, underscoring the need for tailored interventions to support survivors in rebuilding their lives. Expanding the current framework to include longitudinal studies could offer valuable insights into the long-term effectiveness of occupational therapy interventions in promoting sustained recovery and autonomy. Furthermore, prioritising collaboration with interdisciplinary teams and victims/survivors themselves would ensure that future research remains firmly grounded in lived experiences and holistic care approaches. Continuing this line of work will help solidify the evolving role of occupational therapy in addressing intimate partner violence, reinforcing its significance within global health and social care frameworks.

Note

1 The above case study is one of several anonymised examples of individuals who were directly supported through the Domestic Abuse Occupational Therapy Project. In accordance with data protection protocols and to preserve privacy and confidentiality, all identifying information, including names and personal details, has been altered. The inclusion of this case does not require additional consent, as it adheres to professional guidelines for the anonymisation and presentation of data in reflective and academic contexts.

References

Aked, J., Marks, N., Cordon, C., & Thomson, S. (2008, October 22). *Five ways to wellbeing: Communicating the evidence*. Centre for Well-Being/New Economics Foundation. http://neweconomics.org/2008/10/five-ways-to-wellbeing-the-evidence/

Bothelius, K., Kyhle, K., Espie, C.A., & Broman, J.E. (2013). Manual-guided cognitive-behavioral therapy for insomnia delivered by ordinary primary care personnel in general medical practice: A randomized controlled effectiveness trial. *Journal of Sleep Research, 22*(6), 688–696. https://doi.org/10.1111/jsr.12067

Bovend'Eerdt, T., Botell, R., & Wade, D. (2009). Writing SMART rehabilitation goals and achieving goal attainment scaling: A practical guide. *Clinical Rehabilitation, 23*(4), 352–361. https://doi.org/10.1177/0269215508101741

Brown, B. (2015). *Daring greatly: How the courage to be vulnerable transforms the way we live, love, parent, and lead*. Penguin Books.

Clarke, L., & Jones, K. (2021). *Domestic abuse occupational therapy: A project in response to COVID-19*. https://bevancommission.org/domestic-abuse-occupational-therapy-a-project-in-response-to-covid-19/

Critcher, C.R., & Dunning, D. (2015). Self-affirmations provide a broader perspective on self-threat. *Personality & Social Psychology Bulletin, 41*(1), 3–18. https://doi.org/10.1177/0146167214554956

Dixon, A., & Roberts, S. (2013, October 2). *Delivering better services for people with long-term conditions: Building the house of care*. https://www.

kingsfund.org.uk/insight-and-analysis/reports/better-services-people-long-term-conditions

Edhammer, H., Petersson, J., & Strand, S.J.M. (2024). Vulnerability factors of intimate partner violence among victims of partner only and generally violent perpetrators. *Journal of Family Violence*, *39*(2), 235–245. https://doi.org/10.1007/s10896-022-00476-5

Equality and Human Rights Commission. (n.d.). *Domestic abuse is your business*. https://www.equalityhumanrights.com/sites/default/files/da_employers_pack.pdf

Faulkner, S. (2017, June 19–20). *Sleep, sleep problems and sleep treatment: Future directions for occupational therapists*. [Conference session]. 41st Annual Royal College of Occupational Therapists Conference, ICC Birmingham, UK. https://journals.sagepub.com/doi/abs/10.1177/0308022617724785?journalCode=bjod

Forsyth, K., & of Human Occupation Clearinghouse, M. (2006). *A user's manual for the Occupational Circumstances Assessment Interview and Rating Scale (OCAIRS) (version 4.0)*. University of Illinois.

Fritz, H., & Cutchin, M.P. (2016). Integrating the science of habit: Opportunities for occupational therapy. *OTJR: Occupation, Participation and Health*, *36*(2), 92–98. https://doi.org/10.1177/1539449216643307

Fuller, K. (2011). The effectiveness of occupational performance outcome measures within mental health practice. *British Journal of Occupational Therapy*, *74*(8), 399–405. https://doi.org/10.4276/030802211X13125646371004

Hansson, S. O., Björklund Carlstedt, A., & Morville, A. L. (2021). Occupational identity in occupational therapy: A concept analysis. *Scandinavian Journal of Occupational Therapy*, *29*(3), 198–209. https://doi.org/10.1080/11038128.2021.1948608

Helfrich, C.A. (Ed.). (2001). *Domestic abuse across the lifespan: The role of occupational therapy*. Routledge.

Heron, R.L., Eisma, M., & Browne, K. (2022). Why do female domestic violence victims remain in or leave abusive relationships? A qualitative study. *Journal of Aggression, Maltreatment & Trauma*, *31*(5), 677–694. https://doi.org/10.1080/10926771.2021.2019154

Ingram, R.E., & Luxton, D.D. (2005). Vulnerability-stress models. In B.L. Hankin & J.R.Z. Abela (Eds.), *Development of psychopathology: A vulnerability-stress perspective* (pp. 32–46). Sage Publications, Inc. https://doi.org/10.4135/9781452231655.n2

Jones, K. (2020). Bridging the gap. *OTnews*, *28*(8), 54–55. https://www.rcot.co.uk/news/otnews

Kielhofner, G. (2008). *A Model of Human Occupation: theory and application*. 4th ed. Baltimore, MD: Lippincott, Williams and Wilkins.

Kroenke, K., & Spitzer, R. (2002). The PHQ-9: A new depression diagnostic and severity measure. *Psychiatric Annals*, *32*(9), 509–515. https://doi.org/10.3928/0048-5713-20020901-06

Law, M., Baptiste, S., Carswell, A., McColl, M. A., Polatajko, H. J., and Pollock N. (2014). *Canadian occupational performance measure (5th ed.)*. CAOT Publications.

Law, M., Baptiste, S., Carswell, A., McColl, M.A., Polatajko, H.J., & Pollock, N. (2019). *Canadian occupational performance measure* (5th ed. revised.). COPM Inc. https://www.thecopm.ca/

Löwe, B., Decker, O., Müller, S., Brähler, E., Schellberg, D., Herzog, W., & Herzberg, P.Y. (2008). Validation and standardization of the Generalized Anxiety Disorder Screener (GAD-7) in the general population. *Medical Care*, *46*(3), 266–274. https://doi.org/10.1097/MLR.0b013e318160d093

Mattingly, B.A., & Lewandowski, G.W., Jr. (2013). An expanded self is a more capable self: The association between self-concept size and self-efficacy. *Self and Identity*, *12*(6), 621–634. https://doi.org/10.1080/15298868.2012.718863

Monckton-Smith, J. (2023). *What is the homicide timeline?* https://homicide-timeline.co.uk/what-is-the-homicide-timeline.php

Office for National Statistics. (2020). *Domestic abuse in England and Wales: Year ending March 2018*. https://www.ons.gov.uk/peoplepopulationandcommunity/crimeandjustice/bulletins/domesticabuseinenglandandwales/yearendingmarch2018

Oliver, R., Alexander, B., Roe, S., & Wlasny, M. (2019, January). *The economic and social costs of domestic abuse*. UK Home Office. https://assets.publishing.service.gov.uk/government/uploads/system/uploads/attachment_data/file/918897/horr107.pdf

Randal, C., Pratt, D., & Bucci, S. (2015). Mindfulness and self-esteem: A systematic review. *Mindfulness*, *6*(6), 1366–1378. https://psycnet.apa.org/doi/10.1007/s12671-015-0407-6

Rollnick, S., Miller, W.R., & Butler, C.C. (2008). *Motivational interviewing in health care: Helping patients change behavior (applications of motivational interviewing)* (1st ed.). Guilford Press.

Scott, P.J., McKinney, K.G., Perron, J.M., Ruff, E.G., & Smiley, J. (2017). Measurement of participation: The Role Checklist Version 3: Satisfaction and performance. In M. Huri (Ed.), *Occupational therapy – occupation focused holistic practice in rehabilitation* (pp. 107–119). IntechOpen. http://dx.doi.org/10.5772/intechopen.69101

Social Care Institute for Excellence (SCIE). (2022, July). *Co-production in social care: What it is and how to do it*. https://www.scie.org.uk/co-production/what-how/

Taylor, R., Bowyer, P., & Fisher, G. (2023). *Kielhofner's model of human occupation* (6th ed.). Wolters Kluwer.

Twinley, R. (Ed.). (2021). *Illuminating the dark side of occupation: International perspectives from occupational therapy and occupational science*. Routledge. https://doi.org/10.4324/9780429266256

U.S. Centers for Disease Control and Prevention. (2024, May 16). Intimate Partner Violence Prevention: About Intimate Partner Violence. https://www.cdc.gov/intimate-partner-violence/about/index.html

Walker, L.E. (1979). *The battered woman syndrome*. Harper and Row.

Wilcock, A.A. (2002). Reflections on doing, being and becoming. *Australian Occupational Therapy Journal*, *46*(1), 1–11. https://doi.org/10.1046/j.1440-1630.1999.00174.x

Wilcock, A.A. (2006). *An occupational perspective of health*. SLACK.

Women against Abuse. (2025). *The language we use*. https://www.womenagainstabuse.org/education-resources/the-language-we-use

3 Stalking and the role of occupational therapy

Sam Baker

Introduction

Many occupational therapy practitioners pride themselves on being holistic, person centred, and focused on the things that people do that are meaningful and provide value to their everyday lives (RCOT, 2024). Occupations are inextricably linked to our sense of identity and who we are in our society and communities (AOTA, 2024; RCOT, 2024; WFOT, 2024). Occupational therapists work with people day-in, day-out on overcoming barriers to participation and promoting occupations as essential to life and well-being (RCOT, 2024). While these core values and principles demonstrate the power of occupational therapy, in my practice I have experienced that often these values and principles fail to address the full scope of people's engagement in occupation.

I found the dark side of occupation (Twinley & Addidle, 2011, 2012; Twinley, 2021) provided a practical and alternative conceptual lens through which to view and understand occupations; this has been important to me in my practice working with people who have engaged in activities or occupations that have caused harm to both them and to significant others, such as stalking. Working with a criminologist, Twinley and Addidle (2011, 2012) distinctively highlighted how occupations can be deviant or criminal in their nature or form. Such occupations remain overlooked or unexplored within occupational therapy, which has implications for practice. In my practice, I found that stalking is not just unexplored or poorly understood from an occupational perspective; there also remains a significant amount of misinformation; additionally, there is a dearth in understanding from those in criminal justice settings and other relevant professionals. Considering the diverse nature of stalking and the range of behaviours and risk factors, it is understandable that stalking remains an equally significant challenge to the criminal justice system, health, and social care.

Occupations can give lives meaning, purpose, and structure while at the same time causing significant harm, physically or psychologically. Harm can be individual to the person or to significant others or even the wider community and society. This chapter explores the occupation of stalking based on my

DOI: 10.4324/9781032726878-3

professional experience working with perpetrators within England. I highlight how the dark side of occupation is key in developing insight into stalking as an occupation and argue that this perspective and understanding are important in addressing reoffending risk while improving outcomes for victims and communities.

What is stalking?

Stalking can be defined as a "pattern of fixated and obsessive behaviour which is repeated, persistent, intrusive and causes fear of violence or engenders alarm and distress in the victim" (Suzy Lamplugh Trust, 2024). Mullen et al. provide a clinical definition of stalking as: "Repeated attempts to impose unwanted communications and/or contacts on another in a manner that could be expected to cause distress and/or fear in any reasonable person" (2009, p. 10). Historically, stalking has often been thought of as a stranger-based crime where an individual may follow another down a street. It is often presented in television and film material in this manner, and high-profile news outlets frequently present celebrity victims of stalking or harassment. Stalking can happen to anyone, regardless of gender identity, and the course of conduct can be incredibly diverse; for instance, often regarded as a crime involving one victim and one perpetrator, multiple perpetrator stalking also exists, whereby a primary stalker uses other people to further victimise (Logan & Walker, 2017). Stalking and harassment are behaviours that are widely misunderstood (often in the victim's community) and under-reported, yet can cause significant harm to victims, perpetrators, and wider communities (Victorian Law Reform Commission, 2022; McEwan et al., 2017). The diversity of stalking means the crime is highly complex and broad, which leads to a widespread lack of understanding, making it difficult to define from a legal perspective (Crown Prosecution Service [CPS], 2025).

Despite England's introduction of a Stalking Prevention Act in 2019 and its associated Stalking Protection Orders (the guidance for which is issued as statutory guidance under section 12 of the Stalking Prevention Act, 2019), it has had little impact on reducing reoffending or increasing conviction rates. On average it can take victims up to 100 incidents until they report what is occurring to police (Suzy Lamplugh Trust, 2024). In England, only 1.4% of cases reported to police result in a successful prosecution (Suzy Lamplugh Trust, 2023). Low conviction rates combined with misunderstanding lead to significant and long-term impacts on victims of stalking and their families. There is also a notable impact on professionals involved (Harris et al., 2023) and varying motivational factors for the perpetrators themselves who have "diverse psychopathology, characteristic behaviours, and motivations" (British Psychological Society, 2022), which will be explored later in this chapter.

Becoming an occupational therapist in stalking intervention

In 2018, the Multi Agency Stalking Intervention Programme (Jerath et al., 2023) was developed. I joined this programme as the sole occupational therapist, working in one of the three areas of England commissioned by the home office. The aims of the programme were to reduce reoffending rates and improve outcomes for victims. This approach is multi-agency between police, health, probation, and victim advocacy. It is a unique dynamic service and included a unique role for occupational therapy during the pilot phase. This new approach, which diversified from a solely criminal justice response, was identified as the key next step in stalking intervention due to continued low conviction and high reoffending rates.

Stalking can have a significant and life-altering impact on victims. This impact of stalking is as diverse as the behaviour itself, and I feel it is important to explore and highlight this in more depth before illuminating stalking using an occupational lens.

Impact of stalking

Victims/survivors

Stalking has a broad and often catastrophic impact on victims, with the most severe risk being loss of life, either through murder committed by the perpetrator or through suicide by the victim due to the extreme distress caused by stalking (McEwan et al., 2017; Mackenzie et al., 2012; McEwan et al., 2010). The risk of violence increases with closer proximity, as stalking behaviours such as following or accosting are more likely to lead to physical harm than those limited to messaging or phone calls. However, non-physical forms of stalking can still cause severe psychological harm, disrupting daily life, sleep, work, and relationships. Victims may face workplace issues, avoid meaningful activities, and experience social isolation. The diversity of stalking impact is vast and broad and can be devastating to victims. Stalking can lead to serious violence and homicide, and it is important that this level of risk is always considered (McEwan et al., 2017; Mackenzie et al., 2012).

Professionals

While this chapter is not explicitly exploring the specific stalking that targets health and care professionals, it is important to note the risks are like those already described. However, the nature of work in health and social care increases the risk of encountering stalking. This stalking often occurs either from an infatuation for an individual or from a revenge perspective where the perpetrator perceives some form of injustice against them. I have also experienced a case of a health team experiencing stalking as a team, not just a specific individual. The type of risk and potential impact is diverse depending on the typology as previously mentioned, but the nature of working with people who need support with their health and well-being means the risk of encountering this is higher, which can have a significant impact on those working in public services.

Indirect victims/survivors

Stalking not only affects the primary victim, but the research suggests that on average 20 other people are targeted or impacted by stalkers, such as family members, friends, colleagues, or children (Korkodeilou, 2017). Friends and family members will experience the change in behaviour of a victim in distress but also could become victims of stalking themselves. A perpetrator may contact friends or family of a victim to maintain a form of communication, resulting in indirect intrusive behaviours which can have similar impacts. People may also be used unknowingly to facilitate communication with a victim when a perpetrator's means of direct contact are removed. Stalking by proxy is maintained by a third party facilitating communication either knowingly or, more likely, unwittingly. When a third party is used unknowingly in this way and later learns what occurred, there can be an immense sense of guilt and anguish. It can also change a relationship with the victim long term, so the consequences can be far-reaching.

Perpetrators

Crucially, to increase understanding and awareness to protect victims, it is important to understand the impact of stalking on the perpetrators themselves. To do this effectively we must shine a light on the different factors involved in stalking, in the same way the dark side of occupation can shine a light on the whole scope of occupations, which is one reason it aligns with stalking as an intentional behaviour. It may be challenging to acknowledge that stalking can have a significant impact on the perpetrators themselves, but identifying and exploring this are essential to support a more comprehensive and encompassing understanding. This is key in developing effective approaches to reduce risk and recidivism.

Perpetrators engage in stalking for a variety of reasons and motivations (see Table 3.1). Various typology or classification systems exist to support the conceptualisation of stalking behaviour, however none are able to comprehensively explain why people engage in this behaviour (McEwan & Davis, 2020). However, perpetrators always believe they are justified in their pursuit, holding a sense of entitlement. Behaviours escalate and become more

Table 3.1 The different stalking typologies

Typology	*Initial motivation*	*Likely victim(s)*	*Behaviours*	*Risk to victims*	*Occupational factors*
Rejected	Seeking relationship reconciliation or revenge for relationship breakdown	Former sexual intimate partners. Occasionally close family or friends.	Persistent contact, monitoring, and attempts to feel close to the victim or keep the relationship alive. Likely use of third parties as means of communication.	• Emotional distress, potential for escalation to violence, ongoing harassment. • High risk of suicide. • High risk of physical violence.	• Impact on the victim's personal and professional life, loss of focus and productivity. • Low self-esteem and loss of identity for perpetrator. May negate other aspects of life to engage in stalking. • Stalking becomes the sole meaning and purpose for the perpetrator, high risk of suicide or self-harm if this is removed.
Resentful	Perceived injustice from an individual or organisation	Strangers or acquaintances who are seen to have mistreated the stalker. Can be individuals or organisations/ groups.	Stalker may present as the victim, portrays the real victim as an oppressor	• Harassment, psychological harm, potential risk of aggression, often linked to paranoid or delusional beliefs. • High levels of persistence. • Lower risk of physical violence due to lack of proximity, but risk of catastrophic actions escalates over time.	• May affect the stalker's ability to maintain employment or social connections. • Stalkers often significantly socially isolated and withdrawn. • Stalkers likely to have lack of meaningful occupation and limited protective factors. May have experienced occupational deprivation.

(*Continued*)

Table 3.1 (Continued)

Typology	*Initial motivation*	*Likely victim(s)*	*Behaviours*	*Risk to victims*	*Occupational factors*
Incompetent Suitor	Seeking a relationship based on sexual attraction, often due to loneliness or lust	Strangers or acquaintances who the stalker has a sexual attraction to. Motivation is getting a date or short-term sexual relationship.	Unwanted advances, persistent contact, poor awareness of impact on victim Behaviour may be linked to a cognitive deficit or learning disability, but not always	• Psychological harm, risk of ongoing harassment, possible escalation depending on the stalker's persistence. • High risk of recurrence as unable to apply legal boundaries to other people or contexts. • Lower risk of physical violence.	• Difficulty in interpersonal relationships, potential social isolation, and inability to function effectively in social situations. • Likely to have notable skill deficits in communication. • Likely to be experiencing occupational imbalance. • Likely to be socially isolated and find it difficult to build relationships. • Likely to experience occupational deprivation or disruption.
Intimacy Seeking	Desire for an intimate romantic relationship driven by delusional beliefs (erotomania). Wishes to establish emotional connection. This is the only typology where a female perpetrator is more likely.	Strangers or acquaintances become the desire for a long-term relationship.	Persistent stalking due to belief in a destined relationship, fixation on victim. Stalker gains gratification from belief of being closely linked to another.	• High risk of persistent stalking due to mental illness, potential for delusional escalation. • Risk of stalking violence towards third parties, whom the stalker may perceive as 'getting in the way' of the relationship. • Likely to take risks to get close to the victim, including putting self in dangerous situations.	• Impaired social and occupational functioning for both the stalker and the victim, particularly with severe mental illness. • High levels of loneliness. Stalkers will focus solely on this relationship and will negate other aspects of life or other relationships as a result.

(Continued)

Table 3.1 (Continued)

Typology	*Initial motivation*	*Likely victim(s)*	*Behaviours*	*Risk to victims*	*Occupational factors*
Predatory	Motivation to commit a sexual offence. Stalking arises in the context of deviant sexual interests. Stalking maintained by sense of power and control it gives perpetrator.	Usually, female strangers to whom the stalker develops a sexual interest. Stalkers are usually male.	Sexual gratification, initial stalking often covert, victim may be unaware initially. Stalking may be a precursor to a future sexual assault and used to obtain information on the victim.	• High risk of future sexual assault, significant psychological and physical harm to the victim • Impact on the victim's sense of safety, ability to work, and overall quality of life due to fear and trauma.	• Likely to have high levels of skill as covert stalking requires planning, organisation, and abstract thinking. Stalking maintains occupational balance. • Likely to maintaining employment and has a structured daily routine

There are several different stalking typologies used worldwide. The following table is based on the Stalking Risk Profile (MacKenzie et al., 2012). This comprehensive risk assessment is used in the United Kingdom and within multi-agency collaboration to assess risk and understand context behind stalking behaviour (Jerath et al., 2023). It provides a framework for understanding risk related to persistence, recurrence, violence, and risk to the perpetrator themselves. It also guides practitioners in how to work with perpetrators to reduce risk. This table has been adapted to include occupational factors, which have been identified from my work and existing literature on stalking.

intrusive, often lasting a long period of time without effective intervention. Perpetrators will prioritise their stalking behaviours over other elements of their life. This can impact them financially, as they may not pay bills, or they may not attend work and could lose work as a result. They are likely to lose relationships with others, reducing their meaningful social circle. Feelings of loneliness and isolation are highly common within all stalkers and are a key contributor to high levels of recurrence and persistence (MacKenzie et al., 2012; Wheatley, 2019). As the behaviour escalates and other elements of their life are impacted, the stalking becomes the sole priority. They may put themselves at risk of harm in their pursuit of the victim. All these components combined can lead perpetrators to lose financial and relational security alongside losing housing or roles and responsibilities. Those factors may have previously been protective against risk of offending or risk of harm, so in turn stalking becomes their only meaning and purpose. It becomes more intrusive and riskier. If a perpetrator reaches a point whereby they believe they are unable to achieve what they intend to through their stalking, the risk of taking their own life and potentially that of a victim increases exponentially.

Understanding stalking through an occupational lens

Exploring stalking from an occupational perspective entails approaching stalking through an occupational lens. Much work claiming to use an 'occupational lens' does not, however, clarify what that is understood to mean. Adapting Restall et al.'s (2018, p. 185) description of their 'equity lens', I understand an occupational lens to be "a framework to provide a practical starting point for reflecting on" people's occupational experiences. Early on in my stalking intervention practice, I reflected on which occupational therapy constructs and which occupational science concepts were supporting my developing understanding of stalking behaviours. One such concept was occupational balance, which, since engaging with literature for this chapter, has been something I'm more conscious to critically reflect upon.

Contemplating balance and imbalance

As a crime, stalking represents "a unique manifestation of power dynamics and perceived control imbalances for both offenders and victims" (Nobles & Fox, 2013, p. 737). These are problematic patterns of behaviours that both determine and influence the occupations of those engaging in stalking. In this sense, Townsend and Wilcock's (2004) definition of 'occupational imbalance' seemed fitting, considering their depiction of imbalance as constituting a problem due to limited variation in people's occupational engagements. Accordingly, many perspectives have historically asserted the importance of individuals to have a healthy balance between the things we need, want, or are expected to do to promote well-being and enable occupational performance (Eklund et al., 2017; Backman, 2004). Some have argued that definitions of occupational balance do not reflect its complexity (Eklund et al., 2017; Wagman & Håkansson, 2014), suggesting it could be considered as the subjective experience of the balance of occupations within people's own individual lives (Eklund et al., 2017).

Notably, I recognise the very concept has originated from and been mostly studied by scholars from Western societies (Liu et al., 2023). Additionally, the practical utility of occupational balance has been critically reflected upon from the conceptual lens of the dark side of occupation (Cowan & Sørlie, 2021; Dressing et al., 2011). I am mindful of Hammell and Beagan's critical discussion of occupational balance in which they raise concerns, such as "Without a clear conceptualization of what constitutes occupational balance, how might it be determined whether an occupational imbalance exists? . . . If balance – or imbalance – is defined by someone other than the people engaged in the occupations, by what authority does he or she do so, and of what value is his or her opinion?" (2017, p. 61).

In my work, I have found that a consideration of balance is relevant to a stalking population, as those engaging in stalking behaviours often will withdraw from the community or other commitments to continue to pursue their victim.

Within the dynamic risk factors in the aforementioned Stalking Risk Profile, there are a range of lifestyle factors that directly influence recidivism in stalking. Reoffending risk is closely linked to a poorly balanced lifestyle, alongside a lack of, or a reduction in, protective factors. Protective factors are factors unique to an individual that may mitigate or reduce risk (Serin et al., 2016; Mackenzie et al., 2012). These factors can directly influence a perpetrator's occupational balance, highlighting potential areas for occupational therapy intervention (Spitzberg and Veksler (2007); Dressing et al., 2011).

Perpetrators of stalking often have key skill deficits linked to limited educational opportunities during childhood and adolescence and poor social skills linked to individual upbringing (Mackenzie et al., 2012; Dressing et al., 2011). They are often impulsive and can make careless decisions as part of an overall reckless day-to-day life (Spitzberg, 2007; Dressing et al., 2011). Internationally, significant numbers of perpetrators have not completed school education, and many of them lack fundamental skills when it comes to living their daily lives. Mackenzie et al. (2010) found 36% of their sample had completed high school education. Though, when considering such statistics, it is important to consider how there is still a need to codify stalking as a crime in many other countries (Chan & Sheridan, 2020), especially those in the Global South.

This suggests that stalking perpetrators can have a lack of meaning or structure within their everyday life that directly contributes to their engagement in stalking behaviour. Perpetrators often lose meaningful social relationships, job roles, and social engagements because of the pursuit of their victim. I understand this from my perspective as an occupational therapist as being akin to the state of 'occupational imbalance', and this can have long-lasting consequences. The loss of these protective occupations further exacerbates feelings of rejection, resentment, or anger, which then escalates existing stalking. Stalking then can develop from a desire to develop those meaningful relationships, and the pattern of behaviour almost becomes a vocation in itself by providing the meaning, routine, purpose, and structure that paid or unpaid employment could provide. Stalking often then functions to maintain occupational balance, which is why the behaviour persists and escalates over time. Understanding the impact of skills, cognition, and independence of stalking perpetrators is crucial if effective and appropriate treatment options and legal sanctions are to be implemented (Mackenzie et al., 2012). Reoffending rates and risk of recurrence remain high for perpetrators without intervention because they are unable to rebuild some of those fundamental skills, relationships, and meaningful protective factors (Mackenzie et al., 2012).

Stalking is individually complex and can occur in an infinite range of differing contexts (McEwan et al., 2017; MacKenzie et al., 2012). The motivation that underpins stalking might be assessed as a particular typology according to the Stalking Risk Profile, but it remains individually unique for each occurrence. Often this motivation provides such significant meaning that the individual will negate all other factors of their occupational lives to pursue the identified victim (Mackenzie et al., 2012; Spitzberg, 2007). When you consider this, the pattern of behaviour engaged in by a perpetrator provides all the key components of meaningful occupation, namely a specific purpose and intrinsic value (Borell et al., 2022). The vignettes later in the chapter will highlight this issue and identify how occupationally focused intervention can be effective at reducing risk.

A call for an occupational lens

To date, there is no discussion of stalking and stalking-related harassment through an occupational lens in the literature. My role within the multi-agency team was a complex role that combined comprehensive assessment with individual intervention, with the focus of reducing overall reoffending. As the occupational therapist on the team, my primary role was to work with perpetrators on building occupational skills, reintegrating with the wider community and developing strong protective factors to mitigate risk and reduce harm to the perpetrators themselves.

Cronin-Davies (2017) highlights that occupational therapy can support individuals with offending histories to live more purposeful and meaningful lives, develop a more positive sense of identity, increase their protective factors, and thus reduce their overall risk to self, others, and risk of reoffending. Considering that stalking and harassment continue to have high reoffending rates alongside low conviction rates, this strongly highlights that an occupational-based approach could support a potential reduction in risk and help to safeguard victims of stalking. Occupational therapists have a long history of working in forensic settings. The use of occupation to support individuals who have offended recover ordinary lives and improve their well-being leads to reduction in risk and reoffending (RCOT, 2010). It is widely acknowledged that individualised complex interventions are required for stalking perpetrators (Rosenfeld, 2003; James & Farnham, 2003; Mullen et al., 2006; McEwan et al., 2007; McEwan et al., 2009; McEwan et al., 2011; McEwan et al., 2017).

What was the Multi Agency Stalking Intervention Programme?

Prior to exploring real-case scenarios of stalking and occupational therapy practice, I will provide some brief context to the structure and function of the Multi Agency Stalking Intervention Programme. This was and remains a multi-agency team, although its structure has changed in the last few years. During my time in the team, it was a collaboration between health, probation, police, and a victim advocacy service. The overall aim of the programme was to provide an alternate approach to cases of stalking and harassment with the overall purpose to protect victims and reduce recidivism (Jerath et al., 2023).

Referrals into the service would come through a central hub and would be discussed in a multi-agency meeting. Depending on each case, an action plan would be agreed, including direct action by professionals or monitoring, in the case of active criminal investigations. Most referrals came through the police and probation presenting as new cases or individuals with an offending history, with high levels of risk of reoffending. In most scenarios, cases identified that may benefit from health team input (psychology, psychiatry, or occupational therapy) would have an initial assessment with two members of the clinical team. This might involve risk assessment using the stalking risk profile, but it may also be used to ascertain readiness for treatment or to assess mental health components. This information would then be discussed again with multi-agency partners and final action plan agreed. Occupational therapy treatment did not have a specific time date to it but would have specific coproduced goals as outcome measures for progress and changes in risk.

My role in the team also involved using the stalking risk profile to conduct risk assessment to support ongoing criminal investigation as part of a multi-agency panel.

Case vignettes

To illuminate the type of work I was involved in, I provide three case vignettes that outline the salient features of each case, which demonstrate the complexity of stalking and the role of occupational therapy. Each is a different typology of stalking, as described in Table 3.1. To ensure anonymity and protect victims of stalking, names and specific identifiable information have been changed. It is important to note that each of these vignettes is of men as the stalker. During my time in the stalking intervention team, I did not work directly with a woman as perpetrator; the service did encounter a small number of such cases. This aligns with historical and current stalking data and statistics, which is something I will reflect upon at the end of the chapter.

In each case, and through the occupational therapy work described, the Person Environment Occupation Performance (PEOP) model (Baum et al., 2015) was applied as this was useful in providing a structure for occupational analysis for individual cases; in particular, I found, in comparison to many of the traditional occupational therapy models, PEOP provided a structure or understanding of principles linked to the dark side of occupation.

Mr. A, 59 years old (rejected stalker)

Referred to occupational therapy following a joint assessment between psychology alongside his probation officer, Mr. A's stalking behaviour began when his relationship with his girlfriend of two years ended due to reported possessive and controlling behaviour. The behaviour persisted and escalated for two years with intensive unwanted communications through hundreds of daily text messages and phone calls. Despite clear boundary setting by his ex-partner, this communication continued.

When blocked from contacting her via phone and text messages, he sought proximity to her through unwanted contacts. He also followed her in his car and on foot and turned up at her workplace, family member's houses or places she socialised, and used third parties to attempt to contact her, sending messages to family and friends and sending unsolicited gifts as a means of maintaining contact and control.

Despite police intervention and a restraining order, Mr. A's behaviour escalated and culminated with him attempting suicide in view of his ex-partner at her home. This was a non-fatal suicide attempt. Next, he sped on the motorway under the influence of alcohol, which resulted in a two-year prison sentence for stalking, causing the fear of violence.

Mr. A spent most of his time in prison, selectively mute and avoiding interactions with others; he recalled long periods of isolation and occupational deprivation without access to mental health support. Upon release from prison, he was highly resentful and angry over what had happened to him: he perceived that he had been wronged and began taking risks by not adhering to the strict restrictions that were in place with his probation officer.

These restrictions included an exclusion zone in the city where he lived, preventing him from contacting his ex-partner. However, this restriction also prevented him from meeting with *his* friends or participating in previous hobbies or interests. His stalking conviction caused him to lose his job and housing. He had fleeting thoughts of ending his life, and it was clear that he had lost all protective factors. This meant that his risk to self was high, alongside the risk of stalking recurrence, as realistically he had nothing left in his life to lose.

On assessment with occupational therapy, Mr. A was initially very reluctant and somewhat obstructive; he remained angry and resentful and found it difficult to identify goals for the future. Occupational analysis identified the significant loss of protective factors and meaningful occupation as a result of both his stalking behaviour and the occupational deprivation experienced by his release conditions from prison, in place for 12 months and monitored by probation. The initial focus of intervention was on increasing his structure and routine. Initially this involved meeting weekly for a coffee which enabled Mr. A to have a space where he felt heard, understood, and listened to. It also helped to familiarise him with the new area in which he was living while providing a consistent weekly activity to engage in and focus on. This approach of focusing on his occupational identity helped to build trust and rapport which avoided the need to mandate treatment through probation.

Working together, several occupationally focused goals were identified to help Mr. A build protective factors, meaning, and structure into his life:

1. Support Mr. A to seek out more stable and secure housing.
2. Re-engage in employment. He was a high skilled manual worker but had never previously needed to apply for a job using a CV or online platforms. Digital poverty created occupational barriers of a financial nature but also prevented him from working which was a big part of his occupational identity. Low level vocational rehabilitation enabled him to find employment.
3. Engage in leisure occupations. The exclusion zone restricted Mr. A from meeting with friends and taking part in activities such as bridge, pool, and darts. Having a stable place to live enabled him to meet with friends in a new area and I helped him find and identify new locations in which he could take part in his leisure occupations.

Occupational therapy intervention lasted almost six months with weekly 60-minute sessions.

This increase in meaningful occupation supported a shift and change in mindset. Mr. A went from being angry and frustrated at what he perceived as a miscarriage of justice to being reflective and understanding around the impact his behaviour had on other people. His risk of future stalking recurrence was significantly reduced as a direct result of occupational therapy intervention. This was demonstrated through reassessment of the stalking risk profile, and a review following a year of his restrictions being lifted highlighted no further contact or communication had occurred, and the risk remained low.

Mr. B, 28 years old (incompetent suitor)

Referred to the intervention programme following several incidents in a local leisure facility, where he made multiple unwanted contacts with a young female swimming instructor. He approached her and made sexually suggestive comments and contacted the facility asking personal details on several occasions. The final incident occurred when he approached her from behind, grabbed her buttocks in a sexualised manner, and stated he "wanted her to be his girlfriend".

This incident resulted in an arrest and caution for his fifth stalking and harassment offence. Previous legal sanctions for his behaviour had been ineffective. Mr. B had not reoffended against the same victim but had followed a repeat pattern of unwanted and inappropriate communication with multiple other victims.

Despite his ability to obey restraining orders with previous victims, he did not understand that his behaviour was inappropriate and causing harm to others. He was unable to apply information given by police to other social contexts. This suggested a significant social skill deficit consistent with the incompetent suitor typology, whereby stalking and harassment are conducted based on sexual attraction and a desire for relationship. On assessment, Mr. B presented with limited understanding of social norms and was socially isolated. He had very little structure and routine in his life but was highly motivated to avoid further police trouble and engaged well with brief occupational therapy treatment.

Mr. B had a mild learning disability which impacted his understanding of social cues and appropriate behaviour. He had not attended the latter stages of school and spent most of the time with his small family network and had limited support in the community. He had not had the opportunity to develop an understanding of healthy social relationships. He struggled to understand that behaviour deemed to be harmful and inappropriate towards one particular person was also inappropriate and harmful to others too. This was a key factor in his high levels of stalking recurrence over time.

Occupational therapy intervention was brief, with weekly sessions for four weeks. Occupational therapy focused on reducing social isolation and improving social ability to enable Mr. B to participate more actively in society alongside feeling safe and confident in seeking out social relationships with others. This involved behavioural-based interventions, including modelling and developing social stories. Intervention also involved graded exposure to a local community organisation supporting individuals with their mental health; this organisation provided the opportunity to take part in a range of activities in a social environment.

Exposure to this organisation helped Mr. B explore his own occupational identity while also giving him an opportunity to apply and explore his social ability in a supportive environment. Mr B was able to shift his understanding of his behaviour overall rather than direct it towards another. Intervention helped Mr. B understand expectations placed upon him in social situations more clearly. This reduction in social isolation and skill development significantly reduced the risk of future stalking recurrence for Mr. B, and occupational therapy was able to work alongside his support network to provide strategies to support him moving forwards to increase the opportunity to develop healthy relationships with people in the community.

Mr. C, 69 years old (resentful)

Mr. C was referred to occupational therapy to explore meaningful occupations to engage in his post-retirement, and to increase his quality of life and protective factors.

Mr. C's stalking behaviour began with attraction to a healthcare worker but soon became directed towards the local mental health team and council services. It matched behaviours often seen within the rejected typology but was classed under the incompetent suitor, as there was no prior romantic relationship with the healthcare worker. His behaviours included excessive phone calls and letters to her. He would go to her work location asking after her and attempted to leave her unsolicited gifts even after being banned from the location, his care being moved and police warnings. Police action and a restraining order were ineffective at reducing his behaviour.

Mr. C quickly breached his restraining order and followed the healthcare worker to her home and posted letters through the letterbox. This stalking pattern eventually led to another arrest and time spent on remand in prison. Following his release, he continued stalking with a new motivation. He initially made complaints to both mental health teams about his perceived poor treatment and restrictions put on him to protect staff. When the complaints were investigated and dismissed, he began to make complaints to other local authorities and notable figures of a vexatious nature. Despite due process being followed, Mr. C felt he wasn't being listened to, and the organisations were "out to get him". This pattern of stalking led to further criminal justice proceedings, ordering him to attend an assessment with the stalking intervention programme as part of his probation licence. It is important to note that individuals under probation can be court ordered to attend assessments with healthcare professionals, but they cannot be ordered to actively take part in treatment or intervention.

The assessment identified Mr. C as recently retired and socially isolated. He had been a leader in local community which carried importance and responsibility. His occupational identity was heavily tied to his roles of worker, husband, and father. This identity was threatened by his recent loss of regular contact with his adult children and his wife's increasing care needs, which altered his role and purpose in their relationship. They were no longer able to travel with her illness and their income reduction. Mr. C had history of low mood and depression which made him more open to the mental health team. The loss of meaningful roles, leisure occupations, and friendships alongside the changes in his familial relationships left him with a loss of structure and purpose in everyday life which significantly contributed to his stalking.

On assessment, it was identified that his stalking was driven out of a desire to be valued and listened to; he felt that he was not taken seriously by the mental health team, and they had not valued him as an individual. His stalking of the healthcare worker was driven out of a desire for companionship, connection, and sexual attraction. Mr. C misconstrued the healthcare worker's interest in his life as mutual attraction and a desire for a relationship. His social isolation and lack of meaningful occupation led to this search for a relationship and the subsequent search for justice over a perceived mistreatment. The communications and contacts he engaged in provided meaning and structure to his daily routines. Stalking gave him a sense of being valued and part of something – he wanted to take on important leadership-based roles again, and this pattern of behaviour provided some of that to him while at the same time causing significant harm to healthcare staff and his family.

Mr. C refused therapeutic support, so the approach to risk management was to protect victims and utilise appropriate criminal justice processes to reduce the risk of persistence and recurrence. The Stalking Risk Profile identified a range of contributing factors to his offending behaviour within the scope of occupational therapy. Using an occupational lens enhanced the understanding of this behaviour which contributed to the risk management strategies put in place.

Restraining orders were issued for individuals and workplaces with robust risk plans. Mr. C was mandated to work with probation as part of his licence, and specialist training was provided to his probation officer to maintain their boundaries and personal safety. The probation officer set goals to reduce his social isolation and find him meaningful roles. Behavioural contracts were used with his healthcare providers moving forward to ensure appropriate boundaries were maintained and to protect healthcare teams.

Reflection

In writing the above vignettes, I have sought to demonstrate how I used the conceptual lens of the dark side of occupation to support me in understanding the subjective meaning behind stalking, leading to more effective intervention. Having an occupational lens in this area of practice provided a new perspective and approach but also enabled me to re-examine how our theories and models align with the variety of human behaviour.

It is my view that without the encouragement to consider all forms of occupations (as the dark side of occupation concept encourages), we cannot be authentically holistic. It enables us to make a step towards those occupations that remain in the shadows. Be that the shadows of services, behind closed doors, societal oppression, or occupations that we simply have not had the language or structures to effectively understand. Within the context of stalking, the dark side of occupation enables us to understand the subjective meaning behind stalking and stalking-related occupations that people engage in that may be harmful, deviant, health compromising, or poorly understood and ignored. Having this concept, stemming from and relevant to my profession, was like having the agreement for me to drive my unique professional contribution within the team within which I worked.

It is important to reflect that all the included vignettes are of men as perpetrators. During my time within this service, there were very few perpetrators who were women referred through, which is reflective of the statistics on gender and stalking. The data is somewhat outdated, but studies suggest that between 70% and 80% of perpetrators are male (Suzy Lamplugh Trust, 2018; Meloy & Boyd, 2003), and more recently, men were identified as the stalker by women 94% of the time and by men 60% of the time (University of North Carolina at Charlotte, 2023). The exception to this statistic is that of the intimacy-seeking typology, where there is a higher percentage of female perpetrators (Brooks et al., 2021). A standpoint each contributor to this text would uphold is that (much like the issues Bex discusses in Chapter 4) an understanding of stalking perpetrated by women is lacking due to "[r]igid societal beliefs that female-perpetrated crime is not worthy of being taken seriously or is somehow less intrusive has contributed to lower rates of research, reporting, and understanding of female-perpetrated stalking" (Brooks et al., 2021, p. 65). Of additional importance, due to me not having any involvement, the included case vignettes do not represent LGBTIQ+ people who are more likely than heterosexual and cisgender people to experience stalking (Sheridan et al., 2019). Finally, it is critical to recognise that stalking, like other forms of interpersonal violence, is under-reported, and to wonder if there is an even greater occurrence of underreporting when the stalker is a woman.

The dark side of occupation has provided me with the language, understanding, and concept to help understand a complex occupation. It is my view that this has enabled a new perspective and approach to a complex phenomenon. However, despite narrative accounts of the impact of the dark side of occupation existing – many outlined in the Twinley (2021) text – there remains minimal empirical evidence. Hocking and Whiteford (2012) highlight the importance of judging theory and concepts on the impact they have on practice. This is the next step for the dark side of occupation, evidencing the influence it can have on occupational therapy.

Ideas/suggestions for future

- Systematically apply the concepts of the dark side of occupation to stalking behaviours to evaluate the link between theory and practice.
- Continue to disseminate materials using the language of the dark side of occupation to increase awareness and proper use of terminology. I was recently able to present a lecture on the concept in association with the RCOT, which was an important acknowledgement of the relevance of this concept.
- Include discussion and application of the occupation of stalking in occupational therapy/occupational science curricula.
- Conduct research to understand practitioner and educator knowledge and attitudes related to stalking.
- More real-life application of the concept to closer align theory to practice and to follow this up with publications, to share, and to disseminate learning.
- Importance of utilising the correct language (I recently saw an old blog post on social media widely shared on, as they titled it, 'dark occupations', by somebody who has since collaborated with Bex and has discussed the implications of this, such as the harms of prescribing an inherent 'bad' or 'negative' quality to people's occupational choices). This, as I found, ensures we do not stigmatise people through our use of language.
- Hopefully, some of this work can provide arguments for the inclusion of occupational therapy in specialised intervention programmes – an occupational lens should be a core component of such approaches. I would hope this perspective could inform job descriptions or roles in the future.
- Embedding dark side of occupation in occupational therapy education more widely. I believe this provides students with a wider, more comprehensive understanding of occupation.
- Empirical research. I would be particularly keen to see a study on occupational therapists' perspectives of the concept. I often receive feedback on how the concept has changed people's practice, but this is not reflected yet in research.

References

American Occupational Therapy Association (AOTA). (2024). *What is occupational therapy?* https://www.aota.org/about/what-is-ot

Backman, C.L. (2004). Occupational balance: Exploring the relationships among daily occupations and their influence on well-being. *Canadian Journal of Occupational Therapy*, *71*(4), 202–209. https://doi.org/10.1177/000841740407100404

Baum, C.M., Christiansen, C.H., Bass, J.D. (2015). The person-environment-occupation-performance model. In C.H. Christiansen, C.M. Baum & J.D. Bass

(Eds.), *Occupational therapy: Performance, participation and well-being* (4th ed., pp. 49–56). Slack Inc.

Borell, L., Mondaca, M., & Luborsky, M. (2022). "Meaningful occupation" – challenges for occupational therapy research. *Scandinavian Journal of Occupational Therapy, 29*(3), 257–258. https://doi.org/10.1080/11038128.2021.1954996

British Psychological Society. (2022). *Working with individuals who have engaged in stalking: A resource for psychologists.* https://doi.org/10.53841/bpsrep.2022.rep169

Brooks, N., Petherick, W., Kannan, A., Stapleton, P., & Davidson, S. (2021). Understanding female-perpetrated stalking. *Journal of Threat Assessment and Management, 8*(3), 65–76. https://doi.org/10.1037/tam0000162

Chan, H.C.(O.), & Sheridan, L. (Eds.). (2020). *Psycho-criminological approaches to stalking behavior: An international perspective*. John Wiley & Sons Ltd.

Cowan, M., & Sørlie, C. (2021). The dark side of occupation in an eating disorder intensive day service. In R. Twinley (Ed.), *Illuminating the dark side of occupation: International perspectives from occupational therapy and occupational science* (1st ed., pp. 114–121). Routledge. https://doi.org/10.4324/9780429266256-15

Cronin-Davis, J. (2017). Forensic mental health: Creating occupational opportunities. In C. Long, J. Cronin-Davis & D. Cotterill (Eds.), *Occupational therapy evidence in practice for mental health* (2nd ed., pp. 139–164). Wiley-Blackwell. https://doi.org/10.1002/9781119378785.ch7

Crown Prosecution Service. (2025, January 22). *Stalking or harassment.* The Crown Prosecution Service. https://www.cps.gov.uk/legal-guidance/stalking-or-harassment

Dressing, H., Foerster, K., & Gass, P. (2011). Are stalkers disordered or criminal? Thoughts on the psychopathology of stalking. *Psychopathology, 44*(5), 277–282. https://doi.org/10.1159/000325060

Eklund, M., Erlandsson, L.K., Persson, D., & Hagell, P. (2017). The linkage between patterns of daily occupations and occupational balance: Applications within occupational science and occupational therapy practice. *Scandinavian Journal of Occupational Therapy, 24*(1), 41–56. https://doi.org/10.1080/11038128.2016.1224271

Hammell, K.W., & Beagan, B. (2017). Occupational injustice: A critique: L'injustice occupationnelle: Une critique. *Canadian Journal of Occupational Therapy, 84*(1), 58–68. https://doi.org/10.1177/0008417416638858

Harris, N., Sheridan, L., & Robertson, N. (2023). Prevalence and psychosocial impacts of stalking on mental health professionals: A systematic review. *Trauma, Violence, & Abuse, 24*(5), 3265–3279. https://doi.org/10.1177/15248380221129581

Hocking, C., & Whiteford, G.E. (2012). Introduction to critical perspectives in occupational science. In G.E. Whiteford & C. Hocking (Eds.), *Occupational science: Society, inclusion, participation* (pp. 1–7). Wiley. https://doi.org/10.1002/9781118281581.ch1

James, D.V., & Farnham, F.R. (2003). Stalking and serious violence. *The Journal of the American Academy of Psychiatry and the Law, 31*(4), 432–439. https://jaapl.org/content/31/4/432/tab-article-info

Jerath, K., Tompson, L., & Belur, J. (2023). Treating and managing stalking offenders: Findings from a multi-agency clinical intervention. *Psychology, Crime & Law*, ahead-of-print(ahead-of-print), 1–24. https://doi.org/10.1080/1068316X.2022.2057981

Korkodeilou, J. (2017). "No place to hide": Stalking victimisation and its psycho-social effects. *International Review of Victimology, 23*(1), 17–32. https://doi.org/10.1177/0269758016661608

Liu, Y., Wen, S., Zhao, H., & Tan, S. (2023). Occupational harmony: Embracing the complexity of occupational balance. *Journal of Occupational Science, 30*(2), 145–159. https://doi.org/10.1080/14427591.2021.1881592

Logan, T., & Walker, R. (2017). Stalking: A multidimensional framework for assessment and safety planning. *Trauma, Violence, & Abuse, 18*(2), 200–222. https://doi.org/10.1177/1524838015603210

MacKenzie, R.D., James, D.V., McEwan, T.E., Mullen, P.E., & Ogloff, J.R.P. (2010). Stalkers and intelligence: Implications for treatment. *The Journal of Forensic Psychiatry & Psychology, 21*(6), 852–872. https://doi.org/10.1080/14789949.2010.503900

MacKenzie, R.D., McEwan, T.E., Pathe, M., James, D., Ogloff, J., & Mullen, P. (2012). *Stalking risk profile: Guidelines for the assessment and management of stalkers* (2nd ed). StalkInc. & the Centre for Forensic Behavioural Science, Monash University.

McEwan, T.E., Daffern, M., MacKenzie, R.D., & Ogloff, J.R.P. (2017). Risk factors for stalking violence, persistence, and recurrence. *The Journal of Forensic Psychiatry & Psychology, 28*(1), 38–56. https://doi.org/10.1080/14789949.2016.1247188

McEwan, T.E., & Davis, M.R. (2020). Is there a "best" stalking typology?: Parsing the heterogeneity of stalking and stalkers in an Australian sample. In H.C.(O.) Chan & L. Sheridan (Eds.), *Psycho-criminological approaches to stalking behavior: An international perspective* (pp. 115–135). John Wiley & Sons Ltd.

McEwan, T.E., Mullen, P.E., & MacKenzie, R. (2010). Suicide among stalkers. *The Journal of Forensic Psychiatry & Psychology, 21*(4), 514–520. https://doi.org/10.1080/14789940903564370

McEwan, T.E., Mullen, P.E., & Purcell, R. (2007). Identifying risk factors in stalking: A review of current research. *International Journal of Law and Psychiatry, 30*(1), 1–9. https://doi.org/10.1016/j.ijlp.2006.03.005

McEwan, T.E., Mullen, P.E., & MacKenzie, R. (2009). A study of the predictors of persistence in stalking situations. *Law and Human Behavior, 33*(2), 149–158. https://doi.org/10.1007/s10979-008-9141-0

McEwan, T.E., Pathé, M., & Ogloff, J.R.P. (2011). Advances in stalking risk assessment. *Behavioral Sciences & the Law, 29*(2), 180–201. https://doi.org/10.1002/bsl.973

Meloy, J., & Boyd, C. (2003). Female stalkers and their victims. *The Journal of the American Academy of Psychiatry and the Law, 31*(2), 211–219.

Mullen, P.E., Mackenzie, R., Ogloff, J.R.P., Pathé, M., McEwan, T.E., & Purcell, R. (2006). Assessing and managing the risks in the stalking situation. *The Journal of the American Academy of Psychiatry and the Law*, *34*(4), 439–450.

Mullen, P.E., Pathé, M., & Purcell, R. (2009). *Stalkers and their victims* (2nd ed.). Cambridge University Press.

Nobles, M.R., & Fox, K.A. (2013). Assessing stalking behaviors in a control balance theory framework. *Criminal Justice and Behaviour*, *40*(7), 737–762. https://doi.org/10.1177/0093854813475346

Restall, G.J., MacLeod Schroeder, N.J., & Dubé, C.D. (2018). The equity lens for occupational therapy: A program development and evaluation tool: L'Equity Lens for Occupational Therapy: un outil pour le développement et l'évaluation de programme. *Canadian Journal of Occupational Therapy*, *85*(3), 185–195. https://doi.org/10.1177/0008417418756421

Rosenfeld, B. (2003). Recidivism in stalking and obsessional harassment. *Law and Human Behavior*, *27*(3), 251–265. https://doi.org/10.1023/A:1023479706822

Royal College of Occupational Therapists (RCOT). (2010). *Recovering ordinary lives: The strategy for occupational therapy in mental health services 2007–2017: A vision for the next ten years*. College of Occupational Therapists. https://www.rcot.co.uk/sites/default/files/ROL-Vision-for-the-next-10-years_0.pdf

Royal College of Occupational Therapists (RCOT). (2024). *What is occupational therapy?* https://www.rcot.co.uk/about-occupational-therapy/what-is-occupational-therapy

Serin, R.C., Chadwick, N., & Lloyd, C.D. (2016). Dynamic risk and protective factors. *Psychology, Crime & Law*, *22*(1–2), 151–170. https://doi.org/10.1080/1068316X.2015.1112013

Sheridan, L.P., Scott, A.J., & Campbell, A.M. (2019). Perceptions and experiences of intrusive behavior and stalking: Comparing LGBTIQ and heterosexual groups. *Journal of Interpersonal Violence*, *34*(7), 1388–1409. https://doi.org/10.1177/0886260516651313

Spitzberg, B.H., & Veksler, A.E. (2007). The personality of pursuit: Personality attributions of unwanted pursuers and stalkers. *Violence and Victims*, *22*(3), 275–289. https://doi.org/10.1891/088667007780842838

Stalking Prevention Act. (2019). https://www.legislation.gov.uk/ukpga/2019/9

Suzy Lamplugh Trust. (2018). *Myths and realities of stalking*. Suzy Lamplugh Trust. https://www.suzylamplugh.org/Handlers/Download.ashx?IDMF=4fafb4c9-44f5-44bb-8341-a464b89eae84

Suzy Lamplugh Trust. (2023). *An advocate for every victim: Independent Stalking Advocates (ISAs) in the victim and prisoners bill*. https://www.suzylamplugh.org/an-advocate-for-every-victim-independent-stalking-advocates-isas-in-the-victim-and-prisoners-bill

Suzy Lamplugh Trust. (2024). *What is stalking?* https://www.suzylamplugh.org/what-is-stalking

Townsend, E., & Wilcock, A. (2004). Occupational justice. In C.H. Christiansen & E. Townsend (Eds.), *An introduction to occupation: The art and science of living* (pp. 243–273). Prentice Hall.

Twinley, R. (2021). The dark side of occupation: An introduction to the naming, creation, development, and intent of the concept. In R. Twinley (Ed.), *Illuminating the dark side of occupation: International perspectives from occupational therapy and occupational science* (1st ed., pp. 1–14). Routledge. https://doi.org/10.4324/9780429266256

Twinley, R., & Addidle, G. (2011, September 8–9). *Anti-social occupations: Considering the dark side of occupation.* [Conference session]. International Occupational Science Conference: OTs Owning Occupation, Plymouth University, Plymouth, UK.

Twinley, R., & Addidle, G. (2012). Considering violence: The dark side of occupation. *British Journal of Occupational Therapy*, *75*(4), 202–204. https://doi.org/10.4276/030802212X13336366278257

University of North Carolina at Charlotte. (2023, July 18). *Stalking awareness fact sheet – police & public safety.* https://police.charlotte.edu/safety/what-if-i-am-being-stalked/stalking-awareness-fact-sheet/#:~:text=Regardless%20of%20the%20gender%20of,men%2060%20%25%20of%20the%20time

Victorian Law Reform Commission. (2022, September 21). *Stalking: Final report.* https://apo.org.au/node/319642

Wagman, P., Håkansson, C., & Björklund, A. (2012). Occupational balance as used in occupational therapy: a concept analysis. *Scandinavian journal of occupational therapy*, *19*(4), 322–327. https://doi.org/10.3109/11038128.2011.596219

Wheatley, R.C. (2019). *What drives men who commit stalking offences and how practitioners can best respond to their needs (order no. 27766457).* Available from Health Research Premium Collection; ProQuest Dissertations & Theses Global. (2342369477). https://liverpool.idm.oclc.org/login?url=https://www.proquest.com/dissertations-theses/what-drives-men-who-commit-stalking-offences-how/docview/2342369477/se-2

Wheatley, R.C., & Baker, S. (2023). Stalking and the role of occupational therapy "you're not living life to the full if you're stalking". *Journal of Criminal Psychology*, *13*(2), 120–135. https://doi.org/10.1108/JCP-07-2021-0028

World Federation of Occupational Therapists (WFOT). (2024). *About occupational therapy.* https://wfot.org/about/about-occupational-therapy

4 Woman-to-woman rape and sexual assault

Learning from a lesser-known perpetration

Rebecca (Bex) Twinley

Introduction

I start this chapter with my position on rape, which, like all forms of sexual victimisation, I do not exclusively see as a gendered crime. This is in contrast to more traditional perspectives that focus on all forms of interpersonal violence as being deeply rooted in the societal inequalities between women and men. Traditional feminists assert that rape categorically is gendered in nature because statistics report far higher rates of rape victims who are women and perpetrators who are men (Whisnant, 2021). This reinforces many people's perceived need for a focus on man-to-woman perpetration. Undeniably, rape perpetrated by men has harmed women, as a group, and gender-motivated sexual violence against women has long-existed. I myself, as a feminist and a victim/survivor of rape perpetrated by men and women, do not deny man-to-woman perpetration is paradigmatic of patriarchy and misogyny; the very concept of rape and sexual violence is gendered and has its roots in patriarchal societies (Cusmano, 2018). However, disrupting this narrative is necessary if all victims/survivors are to be recognised; acknowledging women as perpetrators will never diminish the harms men have done and continue to do towards women.

Background and my positionality

This discussion is based largely upon my doctoral studies findings, in which I used auto/biography as an epistemological orientation and a (sociological) methodological approach. This compelled me to insert the position of 'I' into my exploration of people's lived experiences that other methods require the researcher to eliminate (Stanley, 1992). Embracing my subjectivity in this way means the 'self' is used as a "resource for helping to make sense of the lives of others [because] it is always present and inseparable from the work we produce" (Letherby, 2003, p. 96).

DOI: 10.4324/9781032726878-4

As a UK-based researcher, the legal context is important to highlight, as this was testified as impacting upon my respondents' post-assault experiences. The UK Sexual Offences Act, 2003, which covers England and Wales, legally defines rape[1] as follows:

(1) A person (A) commits an offence if

  (a) he intentionally penetrates the vagina, anus, or mouth of another person (B) with his penis;
  (b) B does not consent to the penetration;
  (c) A does not reasonably believe that B consents.

Clearly, this heteronormative definition only recognises men as perpetrators of rape and, therefore, excludes women who may, for instance, forcefully penetrate another person. Consequently, this excludes all victims/survivors who have not experienced penile penetration from using the term 'rape' and denies their rights to seeking justice, all of which, in turn, means many experiences are never included in official statistics, audits, or research. Such implications of the legal definition of sexual offences are unfortunately paralleled in several other countries.

Undoubtedly, woman-to-woman rape and sexual assault are very specific forms of sexual perpetration; there are several reasons for my focus on this, as well as implications for practice which I explain hereafter. First, as the person who proposed the theoretical concept of 'the dark side of occupation', providing context to this and the content of this chapter is crucial.

The relevant aspects of my social position are that – at the time I conducted my doctoral research – I identified as a cisgender woman who can be intimately and sexually attracted to other people who self-identify as a woman. Personal experiences of rape and sexual assault by other people – including women – are events that led me to feeling incredibly alone and isolated; finding ways to cope was complex and often maladaptive, which, in turn, contributed to my increasing inability to participate in different aspects of my life. Over ten years after I was raped by a woman during a night out, I found a way to break through some of the silence about this form of perpetration, proposing to conduct my doctoral studies on the issue. Simultaneously, I was experiencing continuing frustration with the restricted lens I perceived was being used to understand and analyse occupations. I felt like the complexity of occupations was not being entirely considered or appreciated. This seemed particularly evident with occupations that are less understood, more stigmatised, or considered 'less acceptable' (often as shared standards of a group of individuals) to be discussed. Consequently, the dark side of occupation was introduced at the time I was engaged in researching adult sexual offending and had been collaborating with a criminology colleague about occupations that are violent and/or criminal (Twinley & Addidle, 2011, 2012).

Woman-to-woman rape and sexual assault: rationale

A key problem is that woman-to-woman rape and sexual assault are real phenomena that globally remain largely unaddressed, as acknowledged by nearly four decades of research in this field (e.g. Brand & Kidd, 1986; Waldner-Haugrud, 1999; Campbell, 2008; Gilroy & Carroll, 2009; Wang, 2011; Walters, 2011; Malinen, 2018; Ovesen, 2023). Official data sources do not capture its prevalence which is further hindered internationally by differing legal definitions of rape and sexual assault. There is acknowledgement that surveys of sexual victimisation which capture rates of the prevalence of women as sexual perpetrators are six times higher than any official data (Cortoni et al., 2017). Due also to limited research endeavours, it is an inadequately understood problem, especially in comparison to rape and sexual assault which is perpetrated by men (Wijkman et al., 2011). Consequently, as I found, victims/survivors cope with little to no support while they endure a range of post-traumatic reactions to the biographical disruption (Bury, 1982) of being sexually victimised (Twinley, 2016).

Setting out to research sexual perpetration others have either never heard of or thought possible was a challenging experience; management of my own emotions and that of others (especially their frustration, disbelief, and assumptions) was at the forefront of the entire endeavour. Over 12 years later, the same problems exist. To illustrate, I return to some of the feedback for Chris's and my proposal for this book. To be clear, we really appreciated our peer reviewer's sharing of thoughts, perspectives, and suggestions and have implemented many valuable recommendations into this text. Some of them did, however, raise some points that may well reflect your own thoughts and which, therefore, Chris and I both felt important to directly respond to, especially related to the content of this chapter. These included (1) 'The focus of woman-to-woman rape/assault seems to disregard IPV (interpersonal violence) among other groups such as gay and transgender persons', (2) 'it is unclear why woman-to-woman rape is an area that would need to be specifically addressed, when the occupational needs of survivors in general have not been adequately addressed', and (3) 'there is and continues to be a plethora of data, worldwide, that rape and sexual assault are gendered in nature. However, that is not to discount the experiences of men as victims of sexual violence'.

To address this feedback, first, gender and sexuality are complex constructs, and the assumption that any research focusing on 'woman to woman' excludes gender and sexually diverse people is inaccurate. I attend to this more in the remainder of this chapter.

Second, I agree, the occupational needs of victims/survivors need to be more adequately addressed. Nonetheless, I contend addressing the occupational needs of victims/survivors "in general" can be informed by research on women as perpetrators (in this case, of other women) just as much as all other forms of perpetration. Concentrating on men as perpetrators of women only reinforces the heteronormativity, heterosexism, and transphobia that is present in, and reinforced by, the predominant evidence base:

> Framing sexual violence as a heteronormative experience, in which men are perpetrators and women are victims, limits recognition and understanding of experiences of sexuality and gender diverse persons (Butler, 1990; Edwards et al., 2015; Griner et al., 2020; Lockwood Harris & Hanchey, 2014; Wooten, 2016).
>
> (Gretgrix & Farmer, 2023, p. 736)

Third, there is "a plethora of data, worldwide, that rape and sexual assault are gendered in nature" because the violence of men against women and femmes has been prioritised while, simultaneously, the violence of women has been silenced or minimised. In actuality, violence has no gender, innately speaking. A colleague who researches women's violence against men explained the implications of sustaining this rigid binary analysis of the gendered nature of sexual violence in their paper with collaborators (Bates et al., 2019). Summarising the relevance of this paper, Gretgrix and Farmer clearly warn others that a rigid view of the gendered nature of sexual perpetration "risks undermining the experiences of victim-survivors who do not fit within 'traditional' gender models or stereotypical expectations, for example individuals who do not identify as male/female or woman/man, non-heterosexuals and/or male victim-survivors" (2023, p. 736). For these reasons, I therefore use my doctoral study on woman-to-woman rape and sexual assault as a case illustration in contrast with the dominance of scholarly works on men's perpetration that rarely applies an intersectional lens.

Study overview

The aim of my doctoral research[2] was to explore the perceived impacts of woman-to-woman rape and sexual assault, the subsequent experience of disclosure, reaction, and support, and the consequences for victims'/survivors' subjective experience of occupation. I therefore sought to illuminate the experience and awareness of woman-to-woman rape and sexual assault among those 159 (adult) members of the world population who responded to a survey, 59 of whom indicated they had experienced a woman sexually assaulting them. Eleven then consented to participating in phase two of my research, sharing their experiences in more depth than the survey permitted; I individually interviewed ten, and an 11th chose to share her story through correspondence. I used the method of thematic analysis to identify, analyse, and report patterns, similarities, themes, and subthemes within the data (Braun & Clarke, 2006). Subsequently, four open themes capturing key aspects of the thematic content from the victims'/survivors' narratives were developed: identity, emotion, survival, and occupation (see Table 4.1).

To explicate, the victims/survivors shared the emotional and deleterious impacts (emotion) which subsequently influenced their subjective experience of occupations (survival). Thus, 47 (80%) of the victim/survivor respondents

Table 4.1 Illustration of the key themes, subthemes, and sub-subthemes identified

Theme	*Subthemes*	*Sub-subthemes*
1. Identity	1.2. Sexual identity	
	1.3. Sexuality	
	1.4. Gender identity	
	1.5. Conceptions of self	1.5.1. As victim/survivor
		1.5.2. As daughter
	1.6. Perpetrator/s identity	
	1.7. Women as sex offenders	
2. Emotion	2.2. Secrecy	
	2.3. Disclosure	
	2.4. Reporting, proof, and justice	
	2.5. Belief and support	
	2.6. Shame	
	2.7. Fear and anger	
	2.8. Hope	
3. Survival	3.2. General health and well-being	
	3.3. Trauma	3.3.1. Coercion, violence, and injury
		3.3.2. Multiple witnesses and perpetrators
	3.4. Mental health and post-traumatic stress disorder	
	3.5. Alcohol use	
	3.6. Self-harm and suicidal behaviour	
	3.7. Accessing support	
4. Occupation	4.2. Daily occupations	
	4.3. Care and restoration	4.3.1. Self-care
		4.3.2. Caring for others
	4.4. Work	4.4.1. Work as triggering and as maintenance
		4.4.2. Could have performed better and achieved more
	4.5. Leisure	
	4.6. Roles and relationships	
	4.7. Alienation and regret (failure to satisfy inner needs)	

felt their victimisation impacted their ability to satisfactorily perform their daily activities, tasks, and things they needed or wanted to do (occupation) linked to their roles and which, therefore, contribute to who they are, their sense of self, and their relationship to others (identity), as their experience of health and of well-being was affected. Next, to provide further insight, I give selected details of each theme, drawing upon illustrative quotes from second-phase respondent data.

As you read this, consider where and how you might knowingly or unknowingly work with a victim/survivor. As an occupational therapist, I wondered about experiences of accessing support or having opportunities to disclose to a health or care professional. I found that only 21 of the 59 victims/survivors did so (none to an occupational therapist), with only ten feeling they received the support they needed. We discuss disclosure, with recommendations, in the final chapter.

Identity

A key issue for the victims/survivors was the negative reactions they received from people they disclosed to. Many recounted their self-perceived ability to even identify as a victim/survivor was thwarted. For all victims/survivors, it is important to understand the 'biographical disruption' (Bury, 1982) brought about by unexpected life events such as rape, which has the potential to either disrupt a person's identity or can trigger a reassessment of their identity and conceptions of self (Hammell, 2004). From the data, I identified two sub-subthemes relating to the latter that represent how the respondents' conceptions of self were impacted, particularly from the perspectives of 1) being a victim/survivor and 2) being a daughter, as I discuss.

Being a victim/survivor

Naming their victimisation experiences was reported as important to the respondents, especially in terms of being able to understand what happened. However, identifying as a 'victim' (especially in the immediate time after the event/s) and, later, for some, as a 'survivor' was challenging, not least because of the silence around woman-to-woman sexual perpetration and its invisibility (especially at the time I conducted the research) in sexual assault support and advice resources and service pathways.

Any route to learning to comprehend what has happened and to manage with the consequences or, even, begin to recover, predominantly starts with the ability to name what has happened. The majority of all survey respondents (38.9%, $n = 23$) named their experience as 'rape'; 32.2% ($n = 19$) named it as 'sexual assault'; 16.9% ($n = 10$) named it as 'sexual violence', with the remaining 13.5% ($n = 8$) naming it as something else, as shown in Table 4.2.

Table 4.2 First phase victim/survivor respondent descriptions used for their sexual victimisation experience/s

Naming your experience	*Number*	*%*
1. Two incidences, first sexual violence, second sexual assault 2. Abuse 3. At the time, I thought it was expected of me to allow this 4. Covert sexual abuse 5. Domestic violence 6. Incident – I can use rape when talking about other peoples, but even as I type this, I feel physically sick 7. Sexual abuse and rape 8. Sexual and manipulative abuse	8	13.5%

Having discussed implications of the lack of legal recognition for woman-to-woman rape and sexual assault victims/survivors in terms of feeling unrecognised and excluded from criminal justice services, respondents also reflected on how others undermined or dismissed their conceptions of self as a victim/survivor. One of the survey respondents who identified as heterosexual and who named their experience rape commented:

> I have received a great deal of invalidation from some people ('friends', etc) who have suggested that the rape I experienced by a woman was at least more 'gentle' and 'less violent' than rape by a man. I have experienced both, and this statement is not true and is very hurtful.
>
> (Survey respondent 156)

Simone, a second-phase respondent, spoke about the lack of validation and associated lack of known places/sources of support to go to when identifying as a woman-to-woman rape and sexual assault victim/survivor:

> [I]n the case of where a woman has been raped by another woman, at the moment, where does she go to say that? Where does a woman go where she feels she can say that? I don't, I can't think of anywhere. I would really like there to be a place.

Being a daughter

In my thesis, I highlight one of the gaps I identified in the existing occupational therapy and science literature (at the time) in terms of the requirement or ability for the victim/survivor to 'be' and 'do' as a daughter. Instinctively, as an occupational scientist, I reflected on Wilcock's developed framework of doing (engagement in meaningful occupations), being (sense of self), and becoming (hopes for the future) (Hitch et al., 2014; Wilcock, 1998, 2006) and the later added belonging (sense of connectedness) (Hitch et al., 2014; Rebeiro et al., 2001). I found the biographical disruption of being sexually victimised influenced their feelings about their role of being a daughter (or child). For Simone and Tanya, this was inextricably linked to the fact that the perpetrator they were each repeatedly victimised by was their own biological mother.

For nine of the respondents, they spoke about contemplating disclosure of their victimisation to family, particularly to their parent/s. However, they reflected on how being a woman with an intimate and/or sexual orientation towards women (Cailey, Eleanor, Isla, Jessica, Kiera, Lauren, and Simone), and/or identifying as transgender (Sarah) or transexual (Ali), had already impacted familial relationships, irrespective of whether or not they were 'out' about this aspect of their identity. This, in turn, meant they anticipated heterosexist, homophobic, or transphobic reactions from their parents or other family members. Additionally, many were aware their performance of their role as daughter had altered, particularly because of their determination to mask or hide things from their parents that had been either affected or created by their victimisation, such as their feelings of safety around women or their increased alcohol use; this masking or hiding was often accomplished through physically and emotionally distancing themselves from their parent/s.

Sexual and gender identity

Discussing these sub-subthemes underscores how there is a crucial need to acknowledge the fluidity of an individual's self-identified and disclosed identity in context (Twinley, 2016); this was certainly essential to understand my respondents' experiences. In terms of sexual and gender identity, Table 4.3 shows the differences in how people self-identify through their responses to my asking, 'How would you describe yourself?' The final column to the right portrays the number of woman-to-woman rape and sexual assault victims/survivors among those respondents that replied to this question.

As raised in Chapter 1, I acknowledged the need to be gender inclusive, which involves being inclusive of trans, non-binary and gender-questioning or diverse people when seeking to recruit respondents who, at the time of their victimisation, identified as a woman who had been raped or sexually assaulted by another woman, or women. As Ghorbanian et al. suggest: "Through the process of acknowledging and validating less visible identities, transgender individuals will be better represented and understood by researchers" (2022, p. 261).

In the second phase of my research, two of the respondents I interviewed identified as 'transsexual' and 'transgender', respectively, Ali and Sarah. When discussing the key theme of identity, gender identity was a prominent

Table 4.3 Survey respondents' self-identified sexual and/or gender identities

How would you describe yourself?	*Number (%) of responses Total N = 159*	*Number of victims/ survivors among these responses*
Bisexual woman	23 (14.6%)	9 (39%)
Gay woman	39 (24.7%)	22 (56%)
Heterosexual woman	42 (26.6%)	7 (16.7%)
Lesbian woman	46 (29.1%)	15 (32.6%)
Free text responses: 1. Asexual, 2. Biological woman, pangender, attracted to women, 3. Bisexual female to male transsexual, 4. Female-bodied trans masculine, 5. Have been bi and gay and straight, 6. Lesbian (without the word "woman"), 7. Queer, 8. Sexual	8 (5.1%)	5 (62.5%)
*No response	1	1

subtheme and crucial to be discussed in relation to Ali and Sarah's stories, especially given the higher levels of sexual victimisation (Truman & Morgan, 2022), lack of regard, insufficient knowledge, and barriers to healthcare for trans and gender-diverse persons (Beagan et al., 2013; Safer et al., 2016). Ali and Sarah both discussed the challenges and transphobia they encountered in relation to their sexuality, sexual, and gender identity. A concern for trans victims/survivors such as Ali and Sarah are the barriers experienced to seeking help in comparison to cisgender people (Howell & Maguire, 2019). In their systematic scoping review, Bach et al. (2021) found sexual assault victims/survivors who identify as gender minorities (including transgender, non-binary, two-spirit) face discrete and, often, additional barriers to accessing and using services. They cite Jordan et al. (2020) who found 'trans-exclusionary' policies at domestic and sexual violence advocacy organisations hinder access. This concern was reported by Ali:

> [Y]ou kind of want to know you can access support if it's been done by a woman and I don't think that's something that's really readily presented . . . the fact that I see what happened as being that kind of sexual assault, I guess it would be kind of nice to also see a sort of representation of trans people as well.

Perpetrator identity

As less is known about woman-to-woman rape and sexual assault, when considering identity, I think it is useful to share who the respondents from the second phase of my research identified as their perpetrator/s. In total, the 11 respondents described 13 instances of rape and sexual assault (Jessica and Simone reported two separate incidences) by a woman. Figure 4.1 shows who the victims/survivors identified their perpetrator/s as. The bottom statistic of 8% represents Sarah's experience, as she was raped by a gang of women and one man, some of whom were known to her and some of whom were not.

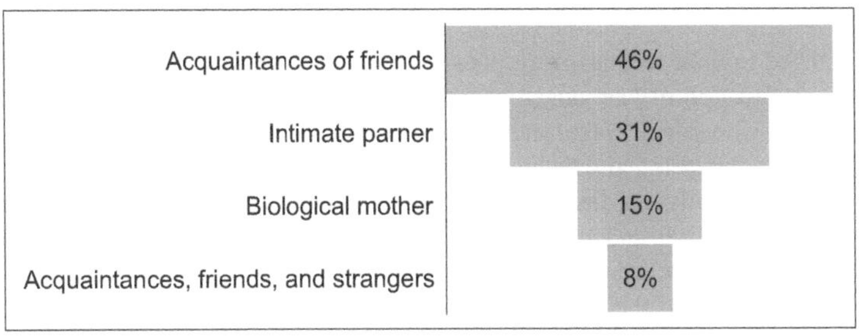

Figure 4.1 Perpetrator identity/relationship to victim/survivor

This data illustrates the range of relationships, pre-existing or not, a woman may have with her/their perpetrator/s. As one of four key themes identified, experiences related to identity – especially in terms of how respondents perceived themselves and expressed and developed their personal identities – are recognised as so significant to their entire daily lived experiences. As Hansson et al. highlight: "The link between occupation and identity is so consequential that an inability to engage in meaningful occupation can threaten identity; similarly, occupation is a means to rebuild one's identity" (2021, p. 198). The destructive impact trauma arising from rape and sexual assault can have on a person's identity correspondingly affects other areas of their lives, such as their experiences of occupations, which are felt in the context of needing to survive, while also enduring its emotional impacts and their subsequent reactions. The next part of this chapter explores this, as I discuss the remaining three key themes that I identified.

Emotion

The magnitude of the short- and long-term emotional impacts of being raped by a woman was such that I reported them through seven identified subthemes of emotion: secrecy; disclosure; reporting, proof, and justice; belief and support; shame; fear and anger; and hope. In relation to fear, and as reported in the literature (Walters, 2011; Wang, 2011; Gilroy & Carroll, 2009; Campbell, 2008; Girshick, 2002), all of the victims/survivors described experiencing fear-based thoughts and feelings immediately and long after their victimisation. The debilitating impacts of living in fear meant their subjective experiences of occupations were affected, often daily:

> I was continually looking over my shoulder for about two years of my life.
>
> (Jessica)

> There was a long time when I was very wary whenever I was in [City] I would – especially if I saw someone in uniform – I would look hard to see if it was her.
>
> (Sarah)

Linked to their feelings of responsibility, every participant told me they felt a combination of fear, anger, or concern for other potential victims, such as Cailey, who stated: "I feel angry about what happened and feel concerned that other young girls and women are going through the same thing".

Additionally, on discussing their feelings and ideas around seeking support, Ali, Lauryn, and Tanya spoke about the hindrance brought about by rape support services and campaigns. Specifically, it was felt that all charities and campaigns focus their efforts primarily upon sexual offences against women and girls perpetrated by men. In particular, one feminist charity was mentioned due to primarily focusing their efforts in this (gendered) way. Their website explains their values under a section headed 'Intersectional feminism', in which they avoid any mention of gender-diverse people or those who identify as trans:

> As a feminist organisation, we fight for equity so that all women and girls can live free from violence and discrimination. . . . We work to understand and address how gender inequality interlinks with other inequalities, including racism, age oppression, class oppression, ableism, homophobia and xenophobia.
>
> (https://rapecrisis.org.uk/about-us/#intersectional-feminism)

For someone such as Tanya, hindrance of their services and campaigns was predominantly experienced in the form of silencing, as Tanya commented:

> These campaigns silence people who have been raped by women. It means they don't come forward. That means because survivors don't come forward society and the people behind these campaigns can go on living with the comfortable idea that women don't rape.

Survival

As respondents reported their post-traumatic reactions, they also described the ways they survived through engagement in occupations – many of which had not, at this time, been sufficiently acknowledged in literature concerning occupations. For instance, the examples below of alcohol use, self-harm, and suicide have received increased attention over the last two decades (Dingus, 2022; Guay et al., 2022; Jennings & Cronin-Davis, 2016; Kirby et al., 2020). Each victim/survivor story of their engagement in such occupations was understood as an example of the human capacity to survive, even though the narrative around victim/survivor coping strategies often cites these as 'negative' or 'maladaptive' (Independent Domestic Abuse Services, 2024; Ullman et al., 2014). This reinforced my use of the term victim/survivor, which describes "the reality of victimisation as well as the fact that the person who is victimised also survives – survives and conquers a crime that society is still unable to deal with effectively" (Taylor, 2004, p. 5).

Survival: alcohol use

Five respondents reported using alcohol following their victimisation which compromised different aspects of their lives, including: 1) their ability to meet self-care and basic daily needs (eating and sleeping), 2) their performance at work, and 3) their participation in sport and exercise. On the latter, Kiera's alcohol use dictated her gym attendance due to not being able to go in the mornings because she would likely still be drunk. Likewise, Simone's sense of belonging to a sports team diminished:

> I used to really like netball. . . . I just stopped going . . . and actually I lost contact with a few of the girls because . . . there was no way I could have told them why I was being the way I was.

Survival: self-harm and suicidal behaviour

Self-harming and suicidal behaviours were experienced either in response to their victimisation – as a means to try to cope – or as a way to express the need for help. For instance, Ali described how he had previously engaged in self-harm which worsened during and after his abusive relationship: 'At the time I was very triggered by it . . . certainly sort of self-harm and stuff sort of escalated. In response to it'. Whereas Cailey described her self-harm as being deliberate and as a purposeful attempt to get help from the teaching staff she felt closest to at the time:

> I went down the route of self-harming in quite a bad way . . . as I've looked back and had counselling and reflected back, I've realised that that was maybe because I wasn't out and I couldn't tell anybody, and so if someone saw that on my arms or on my body – particularly because the people who I related best were the P.E. staff and they would see me in the least clothes – if they noticed that they might be like "What's wrong?" and might be able to save me from it . . . and helped me.

Cailey also declared having suicidal thoughts, and Eleanor and Keira reported suicide attempts. Keira spoke of her suicide attempt as being the catalyst to finding help in the form of a counsellor: 'Once I tried to commit suicide then it was time to live or die, basically, so I thought: Well, if you're going to live, you might as well live a happy life'.

Occupation

Victims/survivors clearly identified that their daily lives and occupations were affected by being raped or sexually assaulted:

> [I]t was almost like the actual impact of it occurred once the relationship was over . . . it does have an ongoing impact on someone's life (Ali).
>
> I think it will always be there. . . . I just think that it will mean that I'm wary of certain situations and certain people forever (Cailey).
>
> I didn't know what normal life was like for everybody else (Eleanor).
>
> it impacted on everything (Isla).

it massively affected my life. . . . I was just really unhappy in all areas of my life really (Jessica).

I could have experienced quite a lot different in life (Keira).

it's dealt with in some ways . . . it still has a bit of an effect (Lauryn).

It's a scar I think, you know? (Sarah).

certainly for me the impact of being raped, both times, was both initial . . . as well as being enduring, you know, it's been a short term and a long term impact on me and my life (Simone).

Now I have to live with the legacy of my abuse that impacts my life every day (Tanya).

Considering this, if we uphold that occupation is "one of the key ways through which people interact, collaborate, communicate and shape their everyday lives together" (Kantartzis, 2019, p. 561), we must realise the ranging and felt effects of being sexually victimised on victims'/survivors' lived experiences. For my respondents, these spanned occupations involving just themselves and involving others, such as sleeping, eating, playing sports, washing and dressing, sex and intimacy, caring for others, working, studying, and socialising in pubs or bars, as the quotes below go some way to illustrate:

> I probably looked very pale and dark eyed because I wasn't sleeping, so that was having an effect on my heath and definitely my wellbeing was just at an all-time low.
>
> (Simone)

> I think it's had a huge effect on how much I trust people. It's only been in the last, maybe in the last couple of years that I've been trusting and more able to speak about things. And just more able to normally interact with people; like I've always been kind of, even when I went to work, not talk about myself at all and people wouldn't know anything about me and I kept things to myself.
>
> (Eleanor)

> I think I've just been a lot more wary about, um, when I'm out and drinks and who I'm with . . . and, you know, ensuring I'm with people I trust more.
>
> (Isla)

> [T]o begin with I think I probably had symptoms of post-traumatic stress right from the outset because, whilst in some people its delayed, um, but I, right from the start I was having nightmares . . . being chased and waking up and feeling like I wanted to scream but I couldn't like my voice had been stolen and I was . . . really hyper vigilant. . . . I was just constantly on alert. . . . I stopped talking to everyone at college and just hid myself in the

> library because I was just, I was scared of everyone and I didn't know what they wanted from me and what their intentions were.
>
> (Lauryn)

Assuming some level of agency and opportunity, it is through daily occupations that individuals can organise their worlds. However, the feelings of disconnection, isolation, hypervigilance, unhappiness, difference, and caution experienced by victims/survivors impede this and, essentially, further deepen the disruption to their everyday subjective experiences of occupations caused by their victimisation.

Evaluation of findings

Respondents' stories reveal the type of impact being raped or sexually assaulted has had upon their subjective experiences of occupations – an issue that demands far more scrutiny from an occupational perspective. The occupational needs of all victims/survivors have yet to be adequately addressed; research endeavours, such as mine, contribute by highlighting types of victim/survivor needs and how these can compromise or influence health, well-being, identity, roles, responsibilities, and connections with others. Victim/survivor occupational needs range from struggling to self-care, making meeting the daily needs of eating and sleeping a challenge, to actively self-harming, which should alert us to the array of things people do in the aftermath of experiencing severe sexual trauma. The issue for those victims/survivors who are further silenced and marginalised by the lack of legal and public address of their form of sexual victimisation (i.e. through exposure to stories or campaigns) is that silence can intensify the impact of trauma (Phillips, 2015; Thomson & Beresford, 2021).

My findings indicate survival reactions and behaviours that I suggest can be understood through applying the conceptual lens of the dark side of occupation, given the need to illuminate and explore many of these occupations from an occupational perspective. For instance, alcohol use, self-harm, and suicidal behaviour are currently under-reported in occupational therapy or science literature (Doğu & Özkan, 2023), particularly subsequent to a traumatic event or experience. This highlights a gap, given the known acute and chronic impact of being sexually victimised includes increased problem use of alcohol (Kirkner et al., 2018), self-harm (Brockdorf et al., 2023), and an increased risk of suicidal thoughts, behaviours, and attempts (Nicholas et al., 2022). Embracing the realisation that occupations are not always health-promoting but may still hold meaning or purpose in people's lives is key to a richer understanding of such engagement (Kjær et al., 2022; Twinley, 2021). An occupational perspective can offer insight into, and explanation of, the altering meaning, role, and nature such occupations have for victims/survivors, in addition to solely concentrating on interventions and recovery.

Implications for practice

Recognition

Primarily, there needs to be far greater recognition that rape and sexual assault can be experienced by any person in any setting; its impacts can be immediate and enduring; and it spans the intersections of age, class, culture, disability, ethnicity, gender identity, migration status, place of residence, race, religion, sex, sexual orientation, and socioeconomic status. This must drive the development of accessible, non-discriminatory, and inclusive frontline services, explicitly promoted to serve the needs of all rape victims/survivors, regardless of these factors, including their gender/identity, or the gender/identity of their perpetrator.

Occupational therapy

As discussed in Chapter 1, there are key reasons why those providing occupational therapy services should be prepared (appropriately trained) to recognise and respond to the needs of sexually victimised people. Occupational therapists are positioned in diverse practice areas where they meet and work with people, groups, and larger populations who, due to their circumstances, can experience limited or unequal occupational opportunities, many of whom will be victims/survivors of some form/s of interpersonal violence. Given how many people experience interpersonal violence in their lifetime, occupational therapists need to be able to understand its effects and manifestations. Any response to the needs of victims/survivors must also be with the awareness that they are at an increased risk of re-victimisation and re-traumatisation. Utilising trauma-informed approaches involves being considerate of a person's "cultural, historical and gender contexts [which] is important as people from different communities may react to trauma differently" (Department for Levelling Up, Housing & Communities, 2023, p. v).

As I found, occupations held great significance in the lives of those victims/survivors who shared their stories with me. Some of these were understood as occupations of and for survival, whereby they were performed to cope or to express their need for support after their victimisation experience/s. Furthermore, their subjective experiences of occupations were shaped by the contrasting contexts in which they were experienced, especially if this was while they were on their own versus being with others, with many sensing an increased alert to the threat of danger when they were alone. This is known as hypervigilance – a persistent PTSD symptom – and can lead to active/deliberate avoidance of certain internal or external reminders of the traumatic incident/s (Bryant, 2019) which, evidently, impedes the individual's occupational performance, participation, and well-being.

I discuss disclosure next but before doing so, I want to acknowledge the complexities of disclosing, talking, and sharing an account of sexual victimisation. I am referring to the intricacies and challenges of deliberating – as a victim/survivor – the question: To tell or not to tell? Not everyone wants to or feels like they can share their story; this does not mean they are any less 'brave' (something I myself have been accused of by a nurse working in a sexual health clinic, sometimes called genitourinary medicine [GUM]) or that they are in any less need of support. Considerations must be made; there are so many factors that silence people or that can place them in a compromised position if they do speak to someone. This can include previous negative disclosure experiences (which could comprise the disclosure being minimised or shaming the victim/survivor), being threatened by the perpetrator (or someone else that knows) to keep quiet, fear of repercussions, including at home or in the workplace, or to a person's work role, and fear of being blamed, let down, or disappointed by the response of the person/s disclosed to.

Disclosure

My respondents echoed the expectation of other sexually victimised people that disclosure will be met by disbelief which invalidates their experiences and decision to disclose (Catton et al., 2023). As eight respondents indicated, a specific barrier to disclosure for sexual and gender-diverse victims/survivors is the fear of being outed or needing to disclose their sexual and/or gender identity and being stigmatised (Edwards et al., 2023). Facilitating disclosure is also met with challenges, as healthcare professionals do not regularly enquire about people's sexual violence history due to a combination of lacking the knowledge, confidence, and skills required to be able to respond appropriately (O'Dwyer et al., 2019). Practitioners need to prepare for, and consider their reactions to, disclosure of rape or sexual assault while, simultaneously, not shaming those who choose not to. Chris and I provide key advice regarding disclosure in Chapter 5.

Additionally, key issues my work in this area has uncovered include the following:

- The human right to justice, including occupational justice, is restricted by the unawareness of woman-to-woman sexual perpetration and the associated lack of address of victim/survivor needs.
- The dark side of occupation can be a useful conceptual lens through which to practically explore difficult, complex, uncomfortable, traumatic experiences, including post-traumatic responses following the experience of being sexually victimised.
- Further research is needed to develop an understanding of the biographical disruption that woman-to-woman (and all other forms of) sexual victimisation can cause to a person's subjective experience of occupation.

Conclusions

I found that woman-to-woman rape- and sexual assault-related post-traumatic survival reactions and behaviours are complex; those that involve victims'/survivors' engagement in lesser understood occupations in order to cope can be recognised from the conceptual perspective of the dark side of occupation. That is, through listening to victims/survivors and by seeking to illuminate their occupations of coping and survival, it is possible to learn about the impact of rape and sexual assault. This impact can be felt immediately, during, or long after victimisation experiences. Indeed, as discussed in Chapter 5, there is no time frame during which the impact on self and on occupations begins or ends. The role of occupational therapists working with victims/survivors and an understanding of how occupations are experienced as people shift from victim to survivor need further illumination.

To summarise this chapter, the discussion of my findings, as represented by the four key themes of identity, emotion, survival, and occupation, illuminates the complexities of the focus of this text; interpersonal violence experiences of rape, sexual assault, stalking, sexual harassment, and intimate partner violence cannot be understood as only cis-gendered men's violence towards cis-gendered women. Woman-to-woman rape and sexual assault remain lesser-known forms of perpetration, and – overall – there is much to learn about woman-to-woman interpersonal violence in terms of the types/forms, tactics, patterns, and intersectional experiences. Given the pervasive and devastating effects of being victimised, service approaches that uphold intersectional principles are crucial, as proficiently explained by Kulkarni (2019, p. 3):

> Intersectional approaches underscore the ways in which social categories, including but not limited to race, class, ability, gender, and sexuality, interact to shape IPV experiences (Potter, 2013; Sokoloff & Dupont, 2005). As a result, individuals contending with multiple oppressions encounter challenges that may or may not be adequately addressed with mainstream IPV services.

I remain aware there are critics who do not agree that women's experiences should, or could, include trans, non-binary, gender-questioning, or gender-diverse people who – at the time/s of their victimisation – have identified as a woman and who perceived their perpetrator to be a woman (as shown in Figure 4.1). Crucially, the issue is that people victimise other people, and the delicate details and intricacies of each case need diligent consideration by those supporting, advocating for, or responding to the needs of the victim/survivor. From the experiences and perspectives of the respondents in my research, the actuality that their perpetrator/s were women influenced much of their subsequent post-traumatic subjective experiences. This can be explained, to some extent, by the very complexities of being able to understand or make sense of the experience of being raped or sexually assaulted by a woman, which is necessary to being able to identify as a victim and/or to even name or recognise the experience as rape or sexual assault.

Interpersonal violence, in all its forms, is a complex problem and one that does not, cannot, rely solely on one means (such as a country's criminal justice system) to try to prevent and respond to the issues it creates. Occupational therapy has a place, much like many other disciplines and professions, in developing non-blaming initiatives, contributing to service improvements, and working as collectives and allies to demand legislative and policy reforms and social and practice changes.

Notes

1 See https://www.legislation.gov.uk/ukpga/2003/42/part/1 for other definitions of offences, such as 'assault be penetration' and 'sexual assault'

2 For full details of methodological approach, please see: Twinley, R. (2016). *The perceived impacts of woman-to-woman rape and sexual assault, and the subsequent experience of disclosure, reaction, and support on victim/survivors' subjective experience of occupation.* [Doctoral dissertation, University of Plymouth] PEARL. https://pearl.plymouth.ac.uk/handle/10026.1/6551

References

Bach, M.H., Beck Hansen, N., Ahrens, C., Nielsen, C.R., Walshe, C., & Hansen, M. (2021). Underserved survivors of sexual assault: A systematic scoping review. *European Journal of Psychotraumatology*, *12*(1), 1895516. https://doi.org/10.1080/20008198.2021.1895516

Bates, E.A., Klement, K.K., Kaye, L.K., & Pennington, C.R. (2019). The impact of gendered stereotypes on perceptions of violence: A commentary. *Sex Roles*, *81*, 34–43. https://doi.org/10.1007/s11199-019-01029-9

Beagan, B.L., Chiasson, A., Fiske, C.A., Forseth, S.D., Hosein, A.C., Myers, M.R., & Stang, J.E. (2013). Working with transgender clients: Learning from physicians and nurses to improve occupational therapy practice: Travailler auprès des clients transgenres: Apprendre des mèdecins et des infirmières en vue d'améliorer la pratique de l'ergothérapie. *Canadian Journal of Occupational Therapy*, *80*(2), 82–91. https://doi.org/10.1177/0008417413484450

Brand, A.P., & Kidd, A.H. (1986). Frequency of physical aggression in heterosexual and female homosexual dyads. *Psychological Reports*, *59*, 1307–1313.

Braun, V., & Clarke, V. (2006). Using thematic analysis in psychology. *Qualitative Research in Psychology*, *3*(2), 77–101.

Brockdorf, A.N., Gratz, K.L., Messman, T.L., & DiLillo, D. (2023). Trauma symptoms and deliberate self-harm among sexual violence survivors:

Examining state emotion regulation and reactivity as dual mechanisms. *Psychology of Violence*, *13*(1), 23–33. https://doi.org/10.1037/vio0000432

Bryant, R.A. (2019). Post-traumatic stress disorder: A state-of-the-art review of evidence and challenges. *World Psychiatry: Official Journal of the World Psychiatric Association (WPA)*, *18*(3), 259–269. https://doi.org/10.1002/wps.20656

Bury, M. (1982). Chronic illness as biographical disruption. *Sociology of Health and Illness*, *4*, 167–182.

Campbell, P.P. (2008). *Sexual violence in the lives of lesbian rape survivors*. [Doctoral dissertation, Saint Louis University, Saint Louis, MO]. Google Books. https://www.google.co.uk/books/edition/Sexual_Violence_in_the_Lives_of_Lesbian/Q87wSAAACAAJ?hl=en

Catton, A.K.H., Dorahy, M.J., & Yogeeswaran, K. (2023). Disclosure of Sexual Victimization: Effects of Invalidation and Shame on Re-Disclosure. *Journal of interpersonal violence*, *38*(13–14), 8332–8356. https://doi.org/10.1177/08862605231155122

Cortoni, F., Babchishin, K.M., & Rat, C. (2017). The proportion of sexual offenders who are female is higher than thought: A meta-analysis. *Criminal Justice and Behavior*, *44*(2), 145–162. https://doi.org/10.1177/0093854816658923

Cusmano, D. (2018). Rape culture rooted in patriarchy, media portrayal, and victim blaming. *Writing across the Curriculum*, *30*. https://digitalcommons.sacredheart.edu/wac_prize/30

Department for Levelling Up, Housing & Communities. (2023, April). *Trauma-informed approaches to supporting people experiencing multiple disadvantage: A rapid evidence assessment*. Crown Copyright. https://assets.publishing.service.gov.uk/media/642af3a77de82b000c31350d/Changing_Futures_Evaluation_-_Trauma_informed_approaches_REA.pdf

Dingus, T. (2022). Expanding knowledge on occupations, one harmful occupation at a time. *Occupation: A Medium of Inquiry for Students, Faculty & Other Practitioners Advocating for Health through Occupational Studies*, *4*(1), Article 1. https://nsuworks.nova.edu/occupation/vol4/iss1/1

Doğu, S.E., & Özkan, E. (2023). The role of occupational therapy in substance use. *Nordisk Alkohol- & Narkotikatidskrift: NAT*, *40*(4), 406–413. https://doi.org/10.1177/14550725221149472

Edwards, K.M., Mauer, V.A., Huff, M., Farquhar-Leicester, A., Sutton, T.E., & Ullman, S.E. (2023). Disclosure of sexual assault among sexual and gender minorities: A systematic literature review. *Trauma, Violence, & Abuse*, *24*(3), 1608–1623. https://doi.org/10.1177/15248380211073842

Ghorbanian, A., Aiello, B., & Staples, J. (2022). Under-representation of transgender identities in research: The limitations of traditional quantitative survey data. *Transgender Health*, *7*(3), 261–269. https://doi.org/10.1089/trgh.2020.0107

Gilroy, P.J., & Carroll, L. (2009). Woman to woman sexual violence. W*omen & Therapy*, *32*, 423–435.

Girshick, L.B. (2002). *Woman-to woman sexual violence: Does she call it rape?* Northeastern University Press.

Gretgrix, E., & Farmer, C. (2023). Heteronormative assumptions and expectations of sexual violence: Language and inclusivity within sexual violence policy in Australian universities. *Sexuality Research and Social Policy*, *20*, 735–750. https://doi.org/10.1007/s13178-022-00718-7

Guay, M., Drolet, M.J., Kühne, N., Talbot-Coulombe, C., & Mortenson, W.B. (2022). What if deliberately dying is an occupation? *The American Journal of Occupational Therapy*, *76*(4), 7604347040. https://doi.org/10.5014/AJOT.2022.047357

Hammell, W.K. (2004). Dimensions of meaning in the occupations of daily life. *Canadian Journal of Occupational Therapy*, *71*(5), 296–305. https://doi.org/10.1177/000841740407100509

Hansson, S.O., Björklund Carlstedt, A., & Morville, A.L. (2021). Occupational identity in occupational therapy: A concept analysis. *Scandinavian Journal of Occupational Therapy*, *29*(3), 198–209. https://doi.org/10.1080/11038128.2021.1948608

Hitch, D., Pépin, G., & Stagnitti, K. (2014). In the footsteps of Wilcock, part two: The interdependent nature of doing, being, becoming, and belonging. *Occupational Therapy in Health Care*, *28*(3), 247–263. https://doi.org/10.3109/07380577.2014.898115

Howell, J., & Maguire, R. (2019). Seeking help when transgender: Exploring the difference in mental and physical health seeking behaviors between transgender and cisgender individuals in Ireland. *The International Journal of Transgenderism*, *20*(4), 421–433. https://doi.org/10.1080/15532739.2019.1658145

Independent Domestic Abuse Services. (2024). *Coping strategies for survivors of sexual assault*. https://sexualviolence.idas.org.uk/surviving-sexual-violence-and-abuse/coping-stategies-for-survivors-of-sexual-assault/

Jennings, H., & Cronin-Davis, J. (2016). Investigating binge drinking using interpretative phenomenological analysis: Occupation for health or harm? *Journal of Occupational Science*, *23*(2), 245–254. https://doi.org/10.1080/14427591.2015.1101387

Jordan, S.P., Mehrotra, G.R., & Fujikawa, K.A. (2020). Mandating inclusion: Critical trans perspectives on domestic and sexual violence advocacy. *Violence against Women*, *26*(6–7), 531–554. https://doi.org/10.1177/1077801219836728

Kantartzis, S. (2019). The Dr Elizabeth Casson Memorial Lecture 2019: Shifting our focus: Fostering the potential of occupation and occupational therapy in a complex world. *British Journal of Occupational Therapy*, *82*(9), 553–566. https://doi.org/10.1177/0308022619864893

Kirby, A.V., Terrill, A.L., Schwartz, A., Henderson, J., Whitaker, B.N., & Kramer, J. (2020). Occupational therapy practitioners' knowledge, comfort, and competence regarding youth suicide. *OTJR: Occupation, Participation and Health*, *40*(4), 270–276. https://doi.org/10.1177/1539449220908577

Kirkner, A., Relyea, M., & Ullman, S.E. (2018). PTSD and problem drinking in relation to seeking mental health and substance use treatment among sexual assault survivors. *Traumatology*, *24*(1), 1–7. https://doi.org/10.1037/trm0000126

Kjær, N.L., Nissen, M.H., Hansen, K.S., Jessen-Winge, C., Sonday, A., & Lee, K. (2022, August 28–31). *Consumption of alcohol as an occupation and the relation to mental health and well-being*. [Conference poster session]. World Federation of Occupational Therapists, Paris, France. https://poster.econference.io/app/wfot/bzxHrTN/poster/100648

Kulkarni, S. (2019). Intersectional trauma-informed Intimate Partner Violence (IPV) services: Narrowing the gap between IPV service delivery and survivor needs. *Journal of Family Violence*, *34*(1), 55–64. https://doi.org/10.1007/s10896-018-0001-5

Letherby, G. (2003). *Feminist Research in Theory and Practice*. Open University Press.

Malinen, K. (2018). Gender, free will, and woman-to-woman sexual assault in service provider discourses. *Affilia*, *33*(1), 56–68. https://doi.org/10.1177/0886109917734497

Nicholas, A., Krysinska, K., & King, K.E. (2022). A rapid review to determine the suicide risk and risk factors of men who are survivors of sexual assault. *Psychiatry Research*, *317*, 114847. https://doi.org/10.1016/j.psychres.2022.114847

O'Dwyer, C., Tarzia, L., Fernbacher, S., & Hegarty, K. (2019). Health professionals' experiences of providing care for women survivors of sexual violence in psychiatric inpatient units. *BMC Health Services Research*, *19*(1), 839. https://doi.org/10.1186/s12913-019-4683-z

Ovesen, N. (2023). Layers of shame: The impact of shame in lesbian and queer victim-survivors' accounts of violence and help-seeking. *Journal of Family Violence*, *39*, 1365–1377. https://doi.org/10.1007/s10896-023-00626-3

Phillips, S.B. (2015). The dangerous role of silence in the relationship between trauma and violence: A group response. *International Journal of Group Psychotherapy*, *65*(1), 65–87. https://doi.org/10.1521/ijgp.2015.65.1.64

Rebeiro, K.L., Day, D., Semeniuk, B., O'Brien, M., & Wilson, B. (2001). Northern initiative for social action: An occupation-based mental health program. *American Journal of Occupational Therapy*, *55*, 493–500. https://doi.org/10.5014/ajot.55.5.493

Safer, J.D., Coleman, E., Feldman, J., Garofalo, R., Hembree, W., Radix, A., & Sevelius, J. (2016). Barriers to healthcare for transgender individuals. *Current Opinion in Endocrinology, Diabetes, and Obesity*, *23*(2), 168–171. https://doi.org/10.1097/MED.0000000000000227

Sexual Offences Act 2003, c, 42. https://www.legislation.gov.uk/ukpga/2003/42/section/1

Stanley, L. (1992). *The auto/biographical I: The theory and practice of feminist auto/biography*. Manchester University Press.

Taylor, S.C. (2004). *Surviving the legal system: A handbook for adult and child sexual assault survivors and their supporters*. Coulomb.

Thomson, S., & Beresford, M. (2021). *Silenced survivors: Understanding gay and bisexual men's experience with sexual violence and support services in the UK*. https://www.survivorsuk.org/wp-content/uploads/2021/07/Silenced-Survivors-A-report-by-SurvivorsUK-.pdf

Truman, J.L., & Morgan, R.E. (2022). *Violent victimization by sexual orientation and gender identity, 2017–2020 (statistical brief)*. US Department of Justice, Bureau of Justice Statistics. https://bjs.ojp.gov/content/pub/pdf/vvsogi1720.pdf

Twinley, R. (2016). *The perceived impacts of woman-to-woman rape and sexual assault, and the subsequent experience of disclosure, reaction, and support on victim/survivors' subjective experience of occupation*. [Doctoral dissertation, University of Plymouth]. PEARL. https://pearl.plymouth.ac.uk/handle/10026.1/6551

Twinley, R. (2021). The dark side of occupation: An introduction to the naming, creation, development, and intent of the concept. In R. Twinley (Ed.), *Illuminating the dark side of occupation: International perspectives from occupational therapy and occupational science* (1st ed., pp. 1–14). Routledge. https://doi.org/10.4324/9780429266256

Twinley, R., & Addidle, G. (2011, September 8–9). *Anti-social occupations: Considering the dark side of occupation*. [Conference presentation]. International Occupational Science Conference: OTs Owning Occupation, Plymouth University, Plymouth, UK.

Twinley, R., & Addidle, G. (2012). Considering violence: The dark side of occupation. *The British Journal of Occupational Therapy*, *75*(4), 202–204. https://doi.org/10.4276/030802212X13336366278257

Ullman, S.E., Peter-Hagene, L.C., & Relyea, M. (2014). Coping, emotion regulation, and self-blame as mediators of sexual abuse and psychological symptoms in adult sexual assault. *Journal of Child Sexual Abuse*, *23*(1), 74–93. https://doi.org/10.1080/10538712.2014.864747

Waldner-Haugrud, L.K. (1999). Sexual coercion in lesbian and gay relationships: A review and critique. *Aggression and Violent Behavior*, *4*(2), 139–149. https://doi.org/10.1016/S1359-1789(97)00054-2

Walters, M.L. (2011). Straighten up and act like a lady: A qualitative study of lesbian survivors of intimate partner violence. *Journal of Gay and Lesbian Social Services*, *23*(2), 250–270. https://doi.org/10.1080/10538720.2011.559148

Wang, Y.W. (2011). Voices from the margin: A case study of a rural lesbian's experience with woman-to-woman sexual violence. *Journal of Lesbian Studies*, *15*(2), 166–175. https://doi.org/10.1080/10894160.2011.521099

Whisnant, R. (2021). Feminist perspectives on rape. In E.N. Zalta & U. Nodelman (Eds.), *The Stanford encyclopedia of philosophy*. Stanford University. https://plato.stanford.edu/entries/feminism-rape/

Wijkman, M., Bijleveld, C., & Hendriks, J. (2011). Female sex offenders: Specialists, generalists and once-only offenders. *The Journal of Sexual Aggression*, *17*(1), 34–45. https://doi.org/10.1080/13552600.2010.540679

Wilcock, A.A. (1998). Occupation for health. *The British Journal of Occupational Therapy*, *61*(8), 340–345. https://doi.org/10.1177/030802269806100801

Wilcock, A.A. (2006). *An occupational perspective of health* (2nd ed.). SLACK Incorporated.

World Federation of Occupational Therapists. (2016). *Minimum standards for the education of occupational therapists*. https://wfot.org/resources/new-minimum-standards-for-the-education-of-occupational-therapists-2016-e-copy

5 Advancing an occupational perspective of interpersonal violence

Rebecca (Bex) Twinley and Christine Helfrich

Introduction

The preceding chapters have illuminated the dark side of occupations involving intimate partner abuse/domestic violence, stalking, and woman-to-woman rape and sexual assault through firsthand accounts of occupational therapists developing programmes, delivering services, and/or conducting research. In these chapters, the respective authors have identified that interpersonal violence is not well defined due to both the diverse nature of the experience and legal definition variation. This results in difficulty discussing, responding to, and penalising these behaviours – all of which leads to grossly inaccurate reports of such crimes. Furthermore, for health and care professionals such as occupational therapists, these issues cause challenges at the point of service access and have consequential challenges with service provision, such as planning and prioritising interventions. Adding to these challenges, victims/survivors are faced with multiple difficulties if they choose to disclose or report to anyone: neither the victim/survivor nor the person they want or need to tell has a common language or understanding. This is magnified with marginalised (as in, underserved) populations where there may also be many gaps in our knowledge and understanding of assault behaviours and cultural barriers which limits how effectively the issue is responded to.

In addition, the discussions in this book highlight that the impact of interpersonal violence can be both short and long term, meaning that the individual is likely to experience immediate as well as long-term consequences resulting from lack of services or secondary or tertiary symptoms that emerge over time. Thus, their recovery may follow a similar pattern where symptoms may not always be immediate and can persist for many years. Despite these complications, occupational therapists have found ways to understand these occupations and have developed promising interventions. The dark side of occupation provides a useful framework to contextualise the lack of understanding and creates permission, if not a mandate, for us to be discussing these issues with our clients and as a profession.

DOI: 10.4324/9781032726878-5

This chapter will synthesise material presented in earlier chapters and outline a direction for the future of practice, research, and education. Although there is much to learn, we know that it is vital to be aware that anyone we encounter may have experienced trauma a long time ago or recently, and it may still be having an impact on them. Victims/survivors may need to work on things in the immediate or longer term. As occupational therapy practitioners and occupational scientists, we must be prepared to hear their stories and guide their occupational explorations. At the very least, all health and care professionals should familiarise themselves with how to respond and what to do if a person discloses that they have been abused (psychologically, physically, sexually, financially, and/or emotionally), harmed, bullied, neglected, coercively controlled, trapped in slavery (including human trafficking), raped, or sexually assaulted.

Appreciating the efforts and legacy of other contributors to this field

The topic of interpersonal violence is high profile across fields such as criminology, social sciences, public health, allied health, social care, medicine, and epidemiology – all of which aim to contribute to an increased and comprehensive understanding of interpersonal violence (van Breen et al., 2024). Contrastingly, we recognise this text is the first of its kind for occupational therapy and occupational science, though we want to emphasise our appreciation for the legacy that other contributors to this small, yet growing collection of literature, have offered. This legacy includes work spanning from childhood to older adults, such as an early study from one of Bex's previous colleagues, Dr Lynda Foulder-Hughes (1998), who examined the education and training needs of occupational therapists who work with adult victims/survivors of childhood sexual abuse, to a student of Chris's who developed a checklist for identifying elder abuse (Lafata & Helfrich, 2001).

More recently, we found a student-produced systematic review aiming to explore the effectiveness of occupational therapy intervention for improving occupational performance for victims/survivors of domestic abuse, published in 2023. In this, they conclude the following:

> [F]uture research should continue to address intervention effectiveness for this marginalized population, and could address the ideal frequency, duration, and specialty intervention within the scope of occupational therapy that would benefit this population.
>
> (Post et al., 2023)

Other works include those in Table 5.1. Please note, this is not an exhaustive list, though it demonstrates the work our colleagues (albeit, predominantly

Table 5.1 Examples of contributions to the field of interpersonal violence from an occupational perspective

Author/s	*Year*	*Full citation*
Ballan et al.	2022	Ballan, M., Freyer, M., & Romanelli, M. (2022). Occupational Functioning among Intimate Partner Violence Survivors with Disabilities: A Retrospective Analysis. *Occupational Therapy in Health Care, 36*(4), 368–390. https://doi.org/10.1080/07380577.2021.1994684
Lynch et al.	2022	Lynch, A., Ashcraft, A., & Tekell, L. (2022). *Trauma, occupation, and participation: Foundations and population considerations in occupational therapy.* AOTA Press. ISBN: 978-1-56900-599-6
Javaherian-Dysinger et al.	2021	Javaherian-Dysinger, H., Dalida, E., Maclang, C., Cho, E., Simbolon, H., & Santiago, M. (2021). Intimate Partner Violence and Occupational Therapy: A Systematic Review. *The American Journal of Occupational Therapy, 75*(S2), 7512520380–7512520380p1. https://doi.org/10.5014/ajot.2021.75S2-PO380
Saleem & Fitzpatrick	2021	Saleem, G.T., Fitzpatrick, J.M. (2021). Impaired Cognition Impacts Occupational Performance and Social Relationships in Survivors of Intimate-Partner-Violence–Related Brain Injury. *The American Journal of Occupational Therapy, 75*(Supplement_2), 7512500071p1. https://doi-org.ezproxy.brighton.ac.uk/10.5014/ajot.2021.75S2-RP71
Humbert et al.	2014	Humbert, T.K., Engleman, K., & Miller, C.E. (2014). Exploring Women's Expectations of Recovery from Intimate Partner Violence: A Phenomenological Study. *Occupational Therapy in Mental Health, 30*(4), 358–380.
Smith & Hilton	2014	Smith, D.L., & Hilton, C.L. (2014). Intimate Partner Violence: Balancing Issues of Identity, Disability Culture, and Occupational Justice to Inform Occupational Therapy Practice. In: D. Pierce. (Ed.) 1st ed., *Occupational Science for Occupational Therapy* (Vol. 1, pp. 157–167). Routledge.
Simpson & Helfrich	2005	Simpson, E.K., & Helfrich, C.A. (2005). Lesbian Survivors of Intimate Partner Violence: Provider Perspectives on Barriers to Accessing Services. *Journal of Gay & Lesbian Social Services, 18*(2), 39–59.
Cooper	2000	Cooper, R.J. (2000). The impact of child abuse on children's play: a conceptual model. *Occupational Therapy International, 7*(4), 259–276. https://doi.org/10.1002/oti.127

(*Continued*)

Table 5.1 (Continued)

Author/s	*Year*	*Full citation*
Foulder-Hughes	1998	Foulder-Hughes, L. (1998). The educational needs of occupational therapists who work with adult survivors of childhood sexual abuse. *British Journal of Occupational Therapy, 61*(2), 68–74. https://doi.org/10.1177/030802269806100205
Davidson	1995	Davidson, D.A. (1995). Physical abuse of preschoolers: identification and intervention through occupational therapy. *The American Journal of Occupational Therapy, 49*(3), 235–243. https://psycnet.apa.org/doi/10.5014/ajot.49.3.235
Froehlich	1992	Froehlich, J. (1992). Occupational therapy interventions with survivors of sexual abuse. *Occupational therapy in health care, 8*(2–3), 1–25. https://doi.org/10.1080/J003v08n02_01
Colman	1975	Colman, W. (1975). Occupational-therapy and child abuse. *The American Journal of Occupational Therapy, 29*(7), 412–417.

from the Global North) have been doing over the past four decades to try to develop and advance our perspective on these issues.

Recommendations for future directions in practice, academia, and research

A notable strength of our writing collaboration is that it was between researcher-academic, practitioner-academic, and professional practitioners. The purpose of this text was to illuminate both the impact of interpersonal violence and the occupational therapy role for practitioners, scholars, educators, and students who are either knowingly or unknowingly working with or alongside victims/survivors. As part of that aim, we sought to provide recommendations for any of the aforementioned when working with people affected by interpersonal violence. Some of these go beyond many local/national policies and procedures the reader will have in place (e.g. safeguarding, lone working, risk assessments). We discuss recommendations in terms of (a) the issue of disclosure, the barriers and facilitators to this, and the potential reasons some victims/survivors choose not to disclose, especially through more formal channels, (b) the application of the dark side of occupation as a conceptual lens to understand the work described, (c) for occupational therapy education/curriculum standards, and (d) for research endeavours.

Revisiting how to talk about interpersonal violence

Recommendations for practice, in particular, but also academia and research, include a consideration of the implications of talking about interpersonal violence. There are likely going to be training needs and concerns for many areas of practice. Addressing interpersonal violence across cultures also highlights contextual variations where, for instance, cultural norms might influence formal service engagement. The sociocultural context can also mean there are disparities in how interpersonal violence is viewed, in its nature, and in its outcomes (Bent-Goodley, 2007). Consider: What have you learned that will enhance your interactions? How will you communicate your openness for people to disclose? What more do you want to learn?

Talking about interpersonal violence necessitates understanding the approaches, referral pathways, and legal frameworks which you can use to support people with whom you work. We would strongly suggest that seeking specialist professional development (such as expert-led and victim/survivor-led or delivered training) regarding interpersonal violence response and prevention activities is both necessary and important. For adults (note, questioning children is different, and you must observe the processes/procedures in your locality), based on a suggestion by West Sussex County Council (n.d.), you could utilise an opening statement like: "As [interpersonal violence/domestic abuse/sexual violence] is so common, we ask everyone who comes to our service if they experience [or have experienced] this. This is because it affects people's safety, health, and wellbeing. We want to ensure we are supporting people and keeping them as safe as possible". In this way, asking the question would be a matter of routine enquiry in your service. Consider that, with any further questioning, in particular, there is the risk that it can be "inappropriate or even harmful to push someone to disclose" (Esposito, 2006, p. 71). Clearly, talking about interpersonal violence in your service/setting warrants much deliberation and specialist support.

Discussing disclosure

Disclosure experiences can either be met with supportive or unhelpful (often, blaming or stigmatising) reactions, leading to varying effects on the victim's/survivor's health and well-being (Edwards & Dardis, 2020; Whitton et al., 2024). For the victim/survivor, there can be much onus on disclosing and, in particular, reporting their victimisation to police or others, especially those working in criminal justice services (advisors and caseworkers). Added pressures to report or disclose involve the insistence to do so to social services (social care), Sexual Assault Referral Centres, a workplace employer, or to other family or community members – all of which can present practical, financial, cultural, and work-related barriers to the victim/survivor, such as loss of earnings, employment, relationships/connections, or home.

Anticipating unsupportive reactions is also a common barrier to disclosure to either close support networks or to formal support/services. Receiving reactions perceived/experienced as unsupportive can lead to more impacts upon mental health, such as post-traumatic stress disorder (Ullman, 2023). Perceptions of reactions and support are crucial to the victim/survivor, as Dworkin et al. (2019, p. 1) explain:

> [P]erceiving social support positively is more important to well-being than the degree to which social support is actually received, and that negative interactions with social supporters are more harmful than positive interactions are helpful.

As a team of occupational therapists, we, as a writing group, recognise the evidence that recommends health and care professionals are generally well placed to encounter victims/survivors through identifying them in their daily work and service provision, yet levels of comfort to raise or discuss interpersonal violence are inconsistent (Heron & Eisma, 2021). For instance, victims/survivors are more likely to need to access health services, and for the older victim/survivor, this need increases as older age groups are most likely to need health and care services; given health professionals work in places where people access and use services, they are in a position to identify older victims/survivors (Macdonald, 2021).

In view of the diverse nature of interpersonal violence perpetration, it is suggested that a victim/survivor-centred approach would place "the rights, wishes, needs, safety, dignity and well-being of the victim/survivor at the centre of all prevention and response measures" (Inter-Agency Standing Committee, 2023). Doing so is intended to ensure the victim's/survivor's safety, security, and well-being are the primary consideration when either informal or formal processes and procedures are being taken in response to any disclosure to avoid them being stigmatised, shamed, or blamed, for example. One recommendation for you, as reader of this text, is to become familiar with disclosure schemes (if you are not already), if they are in place in your geographical locality. In 2014, in the United Kingdom, the government introduced the Domestic Violence Disclosure Scheme (DVDS), also known as 'Clare's Law'. This provides people vulnerable to intimate partner violence (or domestic abuse) access to police records of their partner's criminal (violent) history to be able to make informed decisions. This occurs in one of two ways – either the persons themselves can request information from the police (known as Right to Ask) or police can offer the information (known as Right to Know). Similar schemes are now in place or have been trialled in parts of Australia (New South Wales, Victoria, Queensland), Canada, New Zealand, Northern Ireland, and Scotland. Of note, Clare's Law has been criticised for reinforcing men as perpetrators against women.

When considering issues of disclosure, key advice for health and care professionals from sources such as the Scottish Government (2022, p. 2) recommends the following:

- Respond to disclosure in a trauma-informed, person-centred way, as this is a key step for recovery. Reassure the person that telling you is the right thing to do.
- Never 'interrogate' the person about the incident. If they seem distressed, they may not wish to provide specific details about the incident, and you should not stray into the role of investigator.
- Be alert to the impact on the person of disclosing, perhaps for the first time, whether the events are recent or not.
- Always consider vulnerability and whether the person is an adult who is unable to safeguard their own well-being, property, rights, or other interests; is at risk of harm or is more vulnerable to being harmed because they are affected by disability, mental disorder, illness, or physical or mental infirmity. If so, follow adult support and protection procedures.
- Discuss safety concerns for the person and any children in the household, especially if the perpetrator is known to them. If you know/suspect a child is at risk, follow appropriate child protection procedures.
- Treat any immediate physical or medical condition requiring attention or make necessary arrangements for this.

In addition, regardless of how long after any victimisation experience someone discloses to you, we would recommend the following:

- Be very clear about any limits to, for example, confidentiality and/or any obligations to share information disclosed.
- Listen, avoid interruption, and believe the victim/survivor; reassure them it is not their fault. Validation really matters.
- Never minimise, dismiss, doubt what the victim/survivor discloses, and never try to distract from it (by discouraging speaking further about the victimisation experience) (Lanthier et al., 2018).
- Consider your own beliefs and assumptions and, correspondingly, the language you use. For instance, be aware of damaging gendered narratives that portray men – exclusively – as perpetrators and women as victims/survivors (Widanaralalage et al., 2022). Poor, unhelpful, or negative disclosure experiences can lead to avoidance or delays in disclosing and/or seeking support in the future (Allison et al., 2021) and secondary victimisation.
- Equally, consider the environment within which any disclosure could take place. What messages do display posters or leaflets convey? Who are portrayed as victims and/or as perpetrators? Is there a truly private space away

from anyone attending with the victim/survivor? Does the environment support a culturally competent or appropriate approach to understanding, communicating with, and effectively responding to differing experiences and needs?
- Consider how you frame questions. Explore trauma-informed ways to reframe questions (see, for instance, resource by International Association of Chiefs of Police, 2020) so that you avoid those that inherently blame the victim/survivor, such as any starting with: 'Why didn't you . . .?'
- Provide the necessary information to the victim/survivor, including what you will do in response, clearly outlining the ways to support them, their decisions, and to inform their choices.
- Respect the victim's/survivor's decisions and support their reactions in the aftermath of being victimised.
- For yourself and/or your colleagues, listening to a disclosure can be emotionally distressing; seek and use your internal and external forms of support and find time to debrief and reflect.

Applying the dark side of occupation

As raised in Chapter 1, the dark side of occupation is not the only way to consider complexities of occupations; no single theory or conceptualisation can represent the multifaceted nature of occupations. Its use is not self-fulfilling for Bex, and we encourage readers to always consider alternative lenses – just as each author of this collection does – when engaging critically with the knowledge you acquire, critique, and apply. However, it is, for each of us and many others we have collaborated with, a way to work in what is felt as a valuable, accessible, and authentic way. It is one means through which a critical consideration of many underlying principles of occupational therapy might be challenged or reconsidered, with much of this critique highlighting the binary way in which occupations have, sometimes, been explored or framed.

In Western occupational therapy, there are issues with some of the earlier concepts and frames of reference, such as occupational adaptation, which upholds the perception that people desire to adapt and function, masterfully and effectively, in response to occupational challenges within their environment. Therefore, an adaptive, rather than 'maladaptive', response is proposed as underlying the goals and objectives of the Occupational Adaptation Model when this is applied (Erickson, 2021). There are many implications of such models and, even, of the language they use when applied to victims/survivors of interpersonal violence. The restrictions and barriers to seeking and using adaptive strategies are often overwhelming for the victim/survivor. Whether responses are experienced as adaptive (perceived as 'positive') or maladaptive (perceived as 'negative') can only be determined by the victim/survivor themselves, and use of this binary narrative to describe how people react and respond to challenges or incidents could reinforce feelings of shame and self-blame. The concept of 'mastery' denotes the person must be proficient, effective, and successful in dealing with challenges in their daily lives. For a victim/survivor of interpersonal violence, acts of resistance considered as 'minor' are major strategies that contribute to their survival, often on a day-by-day basis, such as refusing to accept their perpetrator's view of themselves as 'gentle' or 'protecting'.

The imperative value of considering the dark side of occupation in practice and in research is the capacity to explore and illuminate issues people endure that they might not otherwise feel they could discuss, especially with healthcare professionals. This is a task for the profession of occupational therapy in terms of addressing perceptions of what is deemed as 'acceptable', 'tolerable', or 'permitted' to be discussed between a person and their occupational therapist; claiming the provision of holistic or strengths-based practice is questionable if there are occupations people you work with feel they can't discuss, especially those that serve a purpose in terms of helping them to survive or supporting them to achieve some level of coping. Exploring the range of occupations a person subjectively experiences might enhance our understanding of how some can lead people to experience good health but poor states of well-being, and vice versa. If we do not encourage, or even permit, exploration of certain occupations (including those others may perceive or label as unhealthy, maladaptive, or unacceptable), we may be missing the most critical occupations that need to be understood. In the context of the preface of this entire text, occupations of survival are so diverse and distinct and loaded with complexities.

Finally, as has been discussed throughout this book, victims/survivors need to know that what they have experienced is real and worth understanding. Just as children (and adults) need to have racial role models (e.g. Moore et al., 2023) to envision possibilities for themselves, it is similarly important for victims/survivors to know that people like them experience or commit harm and abuse. For example, in Chapter 4, Twinley shares an example of a woman-to-woman rape victim/survivor that did not understand she was raped because the perpetrator was another woman. Describing the occupation of woman-to-woman rape from the perspective of the dark side of occupation validates the victim's/survivor's experience.

Curriculum standards

Many occupational therapy education/curriculum standards of WFOT-approved occupational therapy programmes do not specify any standard considerate of 'trauma', as raised in Chapter 1. The absence of specific standards directly mandating the need to understand trauma across the lifespan results in an absence of such content from most curricula. Despite our own work in this area, we have both had to covertly insert this material into our lectures via research article examples, case studies, or community programme examples.

Just as research endeavours find strengths in co-producing knowledge acquired, standards for occupational therapy education could embrace working in more equal partnerships with victims/survivors and perpetrators, which involves the sharing of power when designing or revising standards.

Research

Research is limited in this area and needs to be expanded despite the challenges and pitfalls in doing so. In a recent conversation between Chris and a student regarding the role of occupational therapy with sexuality, they asked if there was evidence for the programmes discussed. Conducting research on programme effectiveness is expensive and complicated, yet necessary. Occupational science research is doable and will help to further illuminate these occupations which can then be used to provide rationale for experimental studies.

Limitations and associated possibilities

It is our responsibility to identify and discuss limitations of this text and of the perspectives and experiences conveyed within it.

Perpetrator perspectives

Of note, aside from Sam's chapter (Chapter 3), the onus of much of the work described was upon identifying, responding to, and supporting victims/survivors. Equally, in this chapter, we try to consider those providing services and/or working in support services/agencies. Understanding perpetrators of interpersonal violence can improve the ability to respond more effectively and provide adaptable and tailored services to victims/survivors (Hourglass [Safer Ageing], 2024). Moreover, we recognise perpetrator interventions "in most Western societies are based at least in part on feminist ideology in which men's use of violence against women is rooted in patriarchy" (Hine et al., 2022, p. 16) which does not wholly account for all forms of interpersonal violence, particularly that as perpetrated by women. Rather, it is suggested that advancing a more evidence-based and trauma-informed approach that concentrates on the distinctive identified risks and needs of the perpetrator is necessary, especially where traditional intervention approaches have proven ineffective (Barton-Crosby & Hudson, 2021).

Developing a more universal occupational perspective of interpersonal violence

In developing an occupational perspective of interpersonal violence, we undoubtedly recognise there is much need for inclusion and illumination of multicultural, cross-cultural, multilingual, multidisciplinary, diverse, and global perspectives. Occupational therapists should be equipped to demonstrate an understanding of how social categories (e.g. age, class, culture, disability, ethnicity, gender, language, migration status, sexual orientation, race, religion, spirituality, or belief) and a person's or population's unique social and cultural context influence their experiences and reactions to interpersonal violence. Indeed, interpersonal violence can be experienced by any person in any setting; its impacts can be immediate and enduring; and, to reiterate, it spans the intersections of age, class, culture, disability, ethnicity, gender identity, migration status, place of residence, race, religion, sex, sexual orientation, and socioeconomic status. There is a need for, and a possibility of, a future text encompassing broader perspectives and issues related to interpersonal violence experiences; broader than this, as violence manifests in various forms, the role of occupational therapists with victims/survivors of offences/practices such as genital mutilation/cutting, slavery, sexual exploitation, and trafficking warrants examination. Such a text requires great investment of time and care to ensure it inclusively encompasses and centres these diverse and/or minoritised perspectives.

We acknowledge the remit of this 'short form' text was for us (Chris and Bex, as relative scholarly pioneers of interpersonal violence in occupational therapy) to first produce a shorter book, for which the cost would make it more accessible to practitioners and students. We have done so as authors who live and work in Global North countries that have had dominant voices within occupational therapy and, therefore, are not at all reflective of a global perspective. Additionally, this publication can form the basis for any future proposal for an international text. An occupational perspective must deal with the complexities of interpersonal violence, such as (a) those caused and produced by racial disparities, racism, and oppression, (b) the underrepresentation of older victims/survivors among relevant support services, (c) the associations between and ramifications of interpersonal violence for socioeconomic status, including poverty, social exclusion, and homelessness, (d) the links between adverse childhood experiences (ACEs) and increased rates of adult victimisation, (e) the intersection of sexual victimisation, trauma, and (e.g.) autism, or (f) disability-related issues, as discussed next.

Disability-related interpersonal violence

In addition to the points Bex raises in her final thoughts in this chapter, one area we encourage colleagues to pursue and advance an occupational perspective of is the interpersonal violence experiences among disabled people. Researchers from the Center for Research on Women with Disabilities at Baylor College of Medicine (2023) outline how women, for instance, are at increased risk of experiencing unique forms of interpersonal violence that are more likely to occur due to being disabled, such as the following:

> Disability-related Physical Violence – When an abuser physically restrains or confines a person with a disability, handles the person roughly while transferring or assisting in other ways, withholds or destroys their assistive devices (such as wheelchair or cane), withholds their transportation, takes a person in their wheelchair somewhere without their permission, refuses to provide assistance with important personal needs (such as eating or getting out of bed), harms one's service animal, steals or prevents access to prescribed medications. It can also involve taking physical action to prevent a victim from obtaining help for the abuse.
>
> Disability-related Sexual Violence – When an abuser demands or forces sexual activity in return for help, takes advantage of another's physical weakness and inaccessible environment to force sexual activity, or inappropriately touches a person with a disability while assisting with bathing and/or dressing.
>
> Disability-related Emotional Violence – When an abuser rejects or tells a person with disability that they 'deserve' abuse because of their disability, uses disability as an excuse for the abuse, frightens the person by saying they will be sent to an institution if they do not do as told. It can also include making fun of the way a person moves or talks or saying that no one other than the abuser would ever love the person with a disability.

Challenging victim blaming

Victim blaming – whereby blame is partially or entirely transferred from the perpetrator to the victim/survivor – is a significant issue that presents many barriers to the victim's/survivor's potential for accessing support and experiencing some level of recovery. The type of victim blaming can also depend on how different aspects of the victim's/survivor's identity overlap, such as their age, gender, sexuality, race, and disability. In guidance set out to challenge and end victim blaming in the context of violence against women and girls, there is acknowledgement that victims/survivors and perpetrators can span all sexual orientations and gender identities, ages, disabilities, neurodivergences, immigration statuses, races and ethnicities, and religions/spiritualities/beliefs, and cultures. In terms of challenging victim blaming, the guidance suggests:

Practitioners can do this in a constructive and supportive way that encourages people who handle cases to think critically about the potential impact of their language, attitudes, and behaviours. Practitioners should perform the following:

- Challenge harmful stereotypes, assumptions, or jokes that blame victim-survivors for abuse.
- Provide reassurance to victim-survivors that the perpetrator is to blame in their situation, rather than the victim-survivor.
- Hold perpetrators accountable for their actions. Perpetrators will make excuses for their behaviour, but that does not absolve them of what they did.
- In most circumstances, victim-survivors will know what is best for them – support their decision-making wherever possible.
- Recognise that victim blaming is often rooted in discriminatory attitudes or commonly held assumptions which have gone unchallenged.
- Ensure that any written communication and notes remain neutral and are written in a way that does not perpetuate victim blaming (Independent Office for Police Conduct, 2024, p. 9).

Supporting an occupational therapy role in interpersonal violence services

Occupational therapy students, practitioners, and researchers interested in the area of interpersonal violence could study the typologies of interpersonal violence, public health approaches, and the factors that explain why certain people or groups of people are at an increased risk. As Chapters 2–4 have demonstrated, there are many possibilities for occupational therapy roles in the field of interpersonal violence.

There are genuine safety issues for people working to support victims/survivors or perpetrators. Occupational therapists, for instance, might visit the environment/s where violence and abuse are taking place. There are various professional responsibilities and many consequences for a person's emotional and personal safety; witnessing any form of interpersonal violence firsthand can be psychologically detrimental, and engaging empathetically by listening to victims/survivor stories can lead to vicarious trauma (reactions to trauma exposure).

Positionality and emotion work

In discussing safety and bringing this final chapter to a close, we have chosen to return to our positionality, through engaging in reflexivity (a form of critical thinking), to attend to its influence and the negotiation of our insider/outsider/inbetweener positions within the work we each have shared with you. We take a fluid rather than binary approach to being reflexive about our insider/

outsider/inbetweener positionality, as we agree with Milligan (2016) that we (in our roles and from each of our positions) might neither totally be an insider nor an outsider and could operate within a "space between" (Dwyer & Buckle, 2009). This involves disclosure of our 'self' within our work (locating ourselves) to critically reflect on our subjectivities.

Concerning the emotion work

Bex adopted Hochschild's (1983) concept of 'emotion work' in her doctoral studies and, indeed, has continued to do so in her relevant works. Hochschild's (2003/1983) examination of emotion work is about the emotional demands and manipulation of feelings among service-sector employees, whereby it can be necessary to suppress or evoke an emotion. Researching or working in the field of interpersonal violence is emotion work as it involves the management of certain feelings or emotional states. There is also the double burden of conducting this emotion work as emotion when it is often against many of our own colleagues' lack of understanding as to why.

Even in endeavours where others have paved the way, explored the territory, and reflected on its impacts, choosing to enter into the practice of working with or researching victims/survivors of interpersonal violence is a choice fraught with ramifications – personal and professional. Issues of integrity, safety ('theirs' and 'ours'), and ethics are fundamental. Use of supervision and/or other support mechanisms is vital in this work, though not always sufficient, given the complexities of the emotional burden this work can have. Each of us (Kim, Sam, Chris, and Bex) presents some reflections on this here, for the reader.

Kim

Growing up on a council estate (a form of public housing in Britain built by local authorities) where intimate partner abuse was prevalent shaped the course of my life and career. From a young age, I was struck by the prevalence of intimate partner abuse and the profound impact it had on families and communities. However, I often found myself questioning why women stayed in abusive relationships.

I sought to uncover the reasons behind these patterns – why survivors felt unable to leave and why perpetrators behaved one way in private and another in public. As I delved deeper, working with countless women, I began to notice patterns in their stories and behaviours. These were not simply matters of choice but deeply rooted in psychological processes, shaped by thoughts, feelings, and behaviours. This revelation fuelled my desire to learn more and to dedicate my career to addressing these complexities.

In 2020, I became a qualified occupational therapist, an achievement that provided me with new tools and insights for supporting survivors of intimate partner abuse. Occupational therapy offered a fresh perspective – one that focused on helping individuals rebuild their lives through meaningful activities, fostering empowerment, and restoring a sense of identity. I knew that mental health and intimate partner abuse would remain at the heart of my work, as these were the areas where I felt I could make the most impact.

Unfortunately, due to a lack of education and awareness about intimate partner abuse, securing funding to continue my work proved challenging. For a time, I felt compelled to shift my direction, following the opportunities available to me rather than the path I had originally envisioned. Yet my passion for supporting survivors of intimate partner abuse never faded.

It was through Bex's book (Twinley, 2021) and the introduction to Christine and Sam that I rediscovered a sense of connection to the world of intimate partner abuse through occupational therapy. This reignited my passion and reminded me of the importance of addressing intimate partner abuse through a multidisciplinary lens. This collaboration has renewed my commitment to helping survivors rebuild their lives and advocating for the recognition of occupational therapy as an essential part of their recovery journey.

Writing this chapter has allowed me to reflect on my personal and professional journey, becoming a practitioner dedicated to creating meaningful change. I hope my work inspires others to look beyond surface-level judgements and to approach intimate partner abuse with compassion, curiosity, and a commitment to understanding the complex realities survivors face.

Sam

When considering occupational therapy as a potential career choice, I was struck by how much of the promotional material was focused on equipment provision and physical settings. I was enamoured by the concept of occupation but often found myself questioning why the profession was not presented in a more diverse manner or was not more self-critical of its own position. Through the course of my studies and early career, I wanted to push away from this perceived status quo and position myself into different areas which would be challenging but also provide an opportunity to make actual change in terms of pushing the boundaries of the profession and its concepts.

I did not envisage a career that involved so much specialist forensic work, but this work enabled me to actively challenge our core beliefs and structures and learn different perspectives. This was not a straightforward process, and working in both highly secure forensic settings and the stalking service was emotionally demanding. You work – as I did, as an 'outsider' – with individuals who have committed some of the most horrendous acts of violence towards other people, which challenges you as a therapist to maintain objectivity. There have been many times where I have questioned what I am doing, and other people have asked me why I am working with perpetrators. It can be all consuming and dangerous at times. An assault I experienced at the hands of a patient made me question this pathway more than ever. However, what took me back was the belief that nothing changes if we stay in our lanes or do the same things we have always done. I am often critical of occupational therapy for this, as too often we have the same conversations about being misunderstood or not valued, yet not enough is done to challenge these perceptions. Developing an occupational lens of stalking, for example, provided a whole new perspective and treatment approach – and reduced risk. This has a substantial impact on victim safety and the wider community and is a clear demonstration of the power of occupation.

Bex's work connected with me closely as it provided a concept to better understand things I was seeing in practice but did not align with our existing models and structures. By pushing against the tide, I have had experiences and opportunities (such as writing for this book) that I would not have had otherwise, and I am extremely thankful for that.

It's not easy to put your head above the parapet, but that's where real change happens. Don't be afraid of questioning the status quo or stepping into the shadows – you never know what you might find.

Chris

As an occupational therapy practitioner in mental health, I was very aware that the majority of my clients had histories of sexual abuse, as children and/or adults. I was intrigued by the variation in how these histories seemed to impact their current functioning. Reading their histories, observing them in the clinic, and reflecting on my own history made me wonder how I was the treating therapist and not one of the patients myself. Because sexual abuse is hidden in the shadows as something not to be discussed, I refrained from sharing these ideas in supervision or in my graduate work. However, when I began my journey as a PhD student in Public Health, I also began to work on a project for victims of domestic violence (as discussed in Chapter 1) which allowed me to explore these questions from an academic perspective with a child psychiatrist. Listening to children and adults tell their stories of experiencing or witnessing interpersonal violence was difficult. There were days I went home and wrapped myself in a blanket on my couch and talked to no one. As a researcher, I was not able to fulfil my responsibility of documenting everything that happened with a client as fieldnotes. Thankfully, my interviews were recorded, so the integrity of my work was not compromised. When I reached the stage of writing, I was paralysed because I did not want to relive the stories of victimisation and experience all that was stirred up for me in the process. (It is important to note that I was in an immensely helpful therapy relationship and had two academic research supervisors with training to help me manage this work.) Still, I was missing the language and a theoretical perspective to understand why communicating about these topics with others was so difficult. I so wish I had known about the dark side of occupation at that time – communicating the importance of understanding abuse from an occupational science perspective would have been much more manageable with a theoretical framework and language. I am sure that every manuscript and talk would have included these concepts.

Even though I have worked for over three decades developing the role of occupational therapy as discussed in Chapter 1, I realise that editing this book is the first opportunity I have had to discuss and illuminate these issues with other occupational therapy educators, researchers, and practitioners from this perspective, with a shared language. Our profession will not be able to truly embrace our role until we can openly and authentically discuss the dark sides of the occupations discussed in this text. It is my hope that these illuminations of interpersonal violence will provide readers with a framework for further conversation.

Bex

As an 'insider' (i.e. someone who has experienced each form of interpersonal violence this entire text examines), it is comprehensible to realise many of my underlying motivations for wanting to research and write on this topic. Still, motivation alone is never enough to drive the conduct and completion of this work. I needed agreement, for example, to commence my doctoral studies; we needed agreement to author this text for publication. Institutional systems, processes, rules, and expectations are in place that dictate the means and measures people should observe and undergo. Individual team members' thoughts, beliefs, expectations, and values can also dictate or (at the minimum) influence planning this kind of pursuit.

Being silenced as a victim/survivor has led to much self-doubt, self-blame, and feelings of powerlessness, all of which impacted my perception of my choices, whereby I have felt stuck in situations due to feeling like I have no choice. For victims/survivors, this is a place of great vulnerability that can lead to further victimisation or, at the minimum, keep people in harmful or exploitative circumstances due to their vulnerability-related risk. Personally, from vulnerability I have developed great determination, across many aspects of my life. For this reason, I will not, I choose not to, underplay the barriers I felt and had to overcome so that I could research woman-to-woman rape and sexual assault, many of which were communicated in my workplace at that particular point. As a lecturer in occupational therapy, I was fortunate to be able to access a funded place as a part-time PhD student, alongside working in my academic role. However, to gain agreement for what I was going to study,

I had to go outside of my profession and line management, accessing and employing the hierarchical structures in place to my 'advantage' so that a senior signatory would approve my application and proposal. The key reasons I had to do so were because I was told my idea was not 'occupational enough', that I was 'pigeon-holing' (limiting) myself, and that the topic was 'too niche'. I share this because I hope that if any reader also experiences misunderstandings, a lack of understanding, or hostility, they may read this and feel less alone which, in professional terms, can establish interconnectedness and, as a victim/survivor, is a powerful and deeply affirming feeling.

Final thoughts and hopes

Chris

As an occupational therapy and sexuality educator, I am constantly reminded of the challenges for everyone involved to discuss sexuality under any circumstance. These challenges are magnified when the topic or situation involves abuse or maltreatment. When I am providing the Our Whole Lives curriculum (Unitarian Universalist Association, 2025) to children (ages 5–14), my personal goal is to ensure that every child in the class learns two things: first, it is okay to talk about sexual behaviour even if the adult you try to talk to doesn't want to hear it; second, it is never okay to be touched or talked to in a sexual manner that makes you uncomfortable. While the curriculum has many goals, I believe that if participants learn that abuse is not okay, the programme has been successful. Teaching a programme like this requires me to be comfortable discussing so many aspects of occupation that might fall under the concept of the dark side of occupation. My goal is to illuminate these occupations so that they can be understood and destigmatised. It is easier for me to teach and discuss sexuality and identity and orientation with children than with adult learners and colleagues. For example, a good majority of occupational therapy practitioners are not comfortable discussing sexual behaviour, sexual identity, or gender identity (Hwang et al., 2023; Willey et al., 2024). If the practitioner is not comfortable, it is unrealistic to expect them to create an environment for a client to initiate such discussions.

Although our professional organisations have debated the role of occupational therapy with sexuality, the reality is that sexuality is part of the human existence – whether we think it is under our purview or not. Therefore, we must prepare practitioners (and faculty) to be open to discussing sexuality, providing services, and providing referrals as appropriate. Until we can be comfortable discussing consensual intimacy and sexuality, we will never be prepared or competent to address non-consensual or abusive behaviour. Our discomfort in this area is not only invalidating to victims/survivors, but it can also cause harm.

Bex

As a multiply neurodivergent person (autistic, ADHD, living with complex PTSD), I am interested in the genuine development of an occupational perspective and understanding of victimisation experiences so that, for those occupational therapists wanting to develop their knowledge and skills in this area, they are better equipped to understand and apply practical, informed ways of working with people. In terms of neurodivergence, which for many people, such as myself, is experienced largely as a 'hidden disability', there can be additional, distinct barriers and challenges, such as having "difficulty perceiving the true motivation of their abusive" perpetrator and not being "able to discern manipulation or bad intentions as easily as neurotypical victims. Notably, many autistic people 'shut down' when overwhelmed, which creates an additional barrier to help-seeking when experiencing violence" (Lizdas, 2024).

Irrefutably, victims/survivors have unique needs and challenges; both intersectional identities and systemic factors influence victim/survivor experiences, including post-victimisation experiences and the many subsequent decisions they make, such as whether or not to disclose (informally or formally) or to seek support (Cardenas et al., 2024). The pervasive nature of interpersonal violence and its enduring effects are something I cannot ignore. This, therefore, drives me to want to inspire change and advance our occupational perspective in ways that will really impact the way both training/education and practice are delivered and the way inclusive and responsive services are promoted and provided.

Ultimately, I hope those victim/survivor readers of this text take encouragement from the fact there are health and care professionals who genuinely want to do their utmost to support and advocate for your health, well-being, dignity, vulnerability, safety, and rights. My hope includes that any responses you receive incorporate listening, believing, centring you and your experiences, promoting your safety, informing you of your choices, and making you feel assured they seek to respond in the best possible way to your considerations, needs, and challenges that being a victim/survivor of interpersonal violence can cause.

References

Allison, M.K., Marshall, S.A., Stewart, G., Joiner, M., Nash, C., & Stewart, M.K. (2021). Experiences of transgender and gender nonbinary patients in the emergency department and recommendations for health care policy, education, and practice. *The Journal of Emergency Medicine*, *61*(4), 396–405. https://doi.org/10.1016/j.jemermed.2021.04.013

Barton-Crosby, J., & Hudson, N. (2021). *Female perpetrators of intimate partner violence: Stakeholder engagement research.* https://natcen.ac.uk/sites/default/files/2022-12/NatCen_Female-IPV-perpetrators-report.pdf

Baylor College of Medicine. (2023). *Interpersonal violence: Types of interpersonal violence.* https://www.bcm.edu/research/research-centers/center-for-research-on-women-with-disabilities/a-to-z-directory/interpersonal-violence/types-of-interpersonal-violence

Bent-Goodley, T.B. (2007). Health disparities and violence against women: Why and how cultural and societal influences matter. *Trauma, Violence, & Abuse*, *8*(2), 90–104. https://doi.org/10.1177/1524838007301160

Cardenas, I., Graham, L., & Mellinger, M., & Ting, L. (2024). Individuals who experience intimate partner violence and their engagement with the legal system: Critical considerations for agency and power. *Journal of Health Care Law & Policy*, *27*. https://digitalcommons.law.umaryland.edu/jhclp/vol27/iss1/7

Dworkin, E.R., Brill, C.D., & Ullman, S.E. (2019). Social reactions to disclosure of interpersonal violence and psychopathology: A systematic review and meta-analysis. *Clinical Psychology Review*, *72*, 101750. https://doi.org/10.1016/j.cpr.2019.101750

Dwyer, S.C., & Buckle, J.L. (2009). The space between: On being an insider-outsider in qualitative research. *International Journal of Qualitative Methods*, *8*(1), 54–63. https://doi.org/10.1177/160940690900800105

Edwards, K.M., & Dardis, C.M. (2020). Disclosure recipients' social reactions to victims' disclosures of intimate partner violence. *Journal of Interpersonal Violence*, *35*(1–2), 53–76. https://doi.org/10.1177/0886260516681155

Erickson, K. (2021). *Diversity, equity, & inclusion frameworks: A framework for addressing diversity, equity, and inclusion in everyday practice for occupational therapy*. American Occupational Therapy Association. https://www.aota.org/-/media/corporate/files/practice/dei/dei-framework.pdf

Esposito, N. (2006). Women with a history of sexual assault: Health care visits can be reminders of a sexual assault. *American Journal of Nursing*, *106*, 69–73. https://journals.lww.com/ajnonline/citation/2006/03000/women_with_a_history_of_sexual_assault__health.33.aspx

Foulder-Hughes, L. (1998). The educational needs of occupational therapists who work with adult survivors of childhood sexual abuse. *British Journal of Occupational Therapy*, *61*(2), 68–74. https://doi.org/10.1177/030802269806100205

Heron, R.L., & Eisma, M.C. (2021). Barriers and facilitators of disclosing domestic violence to the healthcare service: A systematic review of qualitative research. *Health & Social Care in the Community*, *29*(3), 612–630. https://doi.org/10.1111/hsc.13282

Hine, B., Mackay, J., Baguley, T., Graham-Kevan, N., Cunliffe, M., & Galloway, A. (2022). *Understanding perpetrators of Intimate Partner Violence (IPV)*. https://clok.uclan.ac.uk/32257/1/32257%20Hine%20et%20al.%20VOR.pdf

Hochschild, A.R. (2003/1983). *The managed heart: Commercialization of human feeling*. University of California Press.

Hourglass (Safer Ageing). (2024, September). *Policy brief: Understanding the perpetrators of abuse*. https://wearehourglass.org/sites/default/files/inline-files/Hourglass-Understanding-the-perpetrators-of-abuse.pdf

Hwang, N.K., Park, J.S., & Shim, S.H. (2023). Occupational therapists' views on addressing the sexuality of adult clients in rehabilitation settings:

A qualitative focus group study. *Medicine, 102*(32), e34760. https://doi.org/10.1097/MD.0000000000034760

Independent Office for Police Conduct (IOPC). (2024). *Ending victim blaming in the context of violence against women and girls: Why language, attitudes, and behaviors matter*. IOPC. https://www.policeconduct.gov.uk/sites/default/files/documents/IOPC-ending-victim-blaming-guidance-Feb-2024.pdf

Inter-Agency Standing Committee (IASC). (2023, June 6). *IASC definition & principles of a victim/survivor centered approach*. https://interagencystandingcommittee.org/iasc-champion-protection-sexual-exploitation-and-abuse-and-sexual-harassment/iasc-definition-principles-victimsurvivor-centered-approach-0

International Association of Chiefs of Police. (2020, June 5). *Successful trauma informed victim interviewing*. https://www.theiacp.org/resources/document/successful-trauma-informed-victim-interviewing

Lafata, M.J., & Helfrich, C.A. (2001). The occupational therapy elder abuse checklist. *Occupational Therapy in Mental Health, 16*(3/4), 141–161. https://doi.org/10.1300/J004v16n03_09

Lanthier, S., Du Mont, J., & Mason, R. (2018). Responding to delayed disclosure of sexual assault in health settings: A systematic review. *Trauma, Violence, & Abuse, 19*(3), 251–265. https://doi.org.ezproxy.brighton.ac.uk/10.1177/1524838016659484

Lizdas, K. (2024, June 27). *Neurodiversity and the legal system's response to domestic violence*. https://bwjp.org/neurodiversity-and-the-legal-systems-response-to-domestic-violence/

Macdonald, M. (2021, May 20). *Research briefing: The role of healthcare services in addressing domestic abuse*. House of Commons. https://commonslibrary.parliament.uk/research-briefings/cbp-9233/#:~:text=For%20example%2C%20health%20services%20can,abuse%20than%20non%2Ddisabled%20people

Milligan, L. (2016). Insider-outsider-inbetweener? Researcher positioning, participative methods and cross-cultural educational research. *Compare: A Journal of Comparative and International Education, 46*(2), 235–250. https://doi.org/10.1080/03057925.2014.928510

Moore, C., Coates, E., Watson, A., de Heer, R., McLeod, A., & Prudhomme, A. (2023). "It's important to work with people that look like me": Black patients' preferences for patient-provider race concordance. *Journal of Racial and Ethnic Health Disparities, 10*, 2552–2564. https://doi.org/10.1007/s40615-022-01435-y

Post, M.R., Hohensee, A., Fisher, T., & Malashock, A. (2023). Effectiveness of occupational therapy interventions to enhance occupational performance for survivors of domestic abuse: A systematic review. *Student Systematic Reviews: Occupational Therapy, 8*. https://digitalcommons.unmc.edu/cahp_ot_sysrev/8

Scottish Government. (2022). *Disclosure of rape or sexual assault – guidance document for health care professionals*. Crown Copyright. https://www.gov.scot/publications/sarcs-guidance-healthcare-professionals/documents/

Twinley, R. (Ed.). (2021). *Illuminating the dark side of occupation: International perspectives from occupational therapy and occupational science*. Routledge. https://doi.org/10.4324/9780429266256

Ullman, S.E. (2023). Correlates of social reactions to victims' disclosures of sexual assault and intimate partner violence: A systematic review. *Trauma, Violence, & Abuse*, *24*(1), 29–43. https://doi.org/10.1177/15248380211016013

Unitarian Universalist Association. (2025, January 30). *Our whole lives: Lifespan sexuality education*. Our Whole Lives: Lifespan Sexuality Education | UUA.org

van Breen, J., Kivivuori, J., Nivette, A., Kiefte-de Jong, J., Liem, M., & on behalf of the Interpersonal Violence Consortium. (2024). The future of interpersonal violence research: Steps towards interdisciplinary integration. *Humanities & Social Sciences Communications*, *11*(1), 1303–1307. https://doi.org/10.1057/s41599-024-03760-5

West Sussex County Council. (n.d.). *Domestic abuse home: Professionals working with victim-survivors*. https://www.westsussex.gov.uk/fire-emergencies-and-crime/domestic-abuse/professionals-working-with-victim-survivors/

Whitton, S.W., Devlin, E.A., Lawlace, M., & Newcomb, M.E. (2024). Disclosure and help-seeking experiences of sexual and gender minority victims of intimate partner violence: A mixed-methods study. *Journal of Interpersonal Violence*, *39*(7–8), 1373–1397. https://doi.org/10.1177/08862605231207618

Widanaralalage, B.K., Hine, B.A., Murphy, A.D., & Murji, K. (2022). "I didn't feel I was a victim": A phenomenological analysis of the experiences of male-on-male survivors of rape and sexual abuse. *Victims & Offenders*, *17*(8), 1147–1172. https://doi.org/10.1080/15564886.2022.2069898

Willey, K.S., Howell, D., & Skubik-Peplaski, C. (2024). Occupational therapists' consideration of sexual orientation and gender identity when working with adolescents: A preliminary study. *The Open Journal of Occupational Therapy*, *12*(3), 1–10. https://doi.org/10.15453/2168–6408.2202

Index